KE1
THE 100-CALORIE
STEPLADDER TO
SUCCESS

Some, as thou saw'st, by violent stroke shall die,
By fire, flood, famine, by intemperance more
In meats and drinks which on earth shall bring diseases dire.

John Milton, *Paradise Lost*, Book 11, lines 471-474

KETOFAST:
THE 100-CALORIE
STEPLADDER TO
SUCCESS

BY

LARRY S. MILNER, M.D.

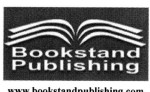

www.bookstandpublishing.com

Published by
Bookstand Publishing
Morgan Hill, CA 95037
3128_2

ISBN 978-1-58909-723-0

Printed in the United States of America

TABLE OF CONTENTS

TABLE OF CONTENTS (Concluded)

I. INTRODUCTION

This book may save your life, or the life of a loved one.

I do not make this claim lightly, and my intention is not to relegate myself to the level of a sideshow barker, but I want to emphasize at the very outset of this book how dangerous obesity is to your health. I realize you have probably heard this message before, *ad infinitum*, from family, friends, and physicians during your multiple attempts to diet with only partial or temporary success. You may have even given up hope that you can ever change the way you are, and decided instead that the stress and strain on your body from repetitive failures of diet programs is not worth the effort you have put forth. Well, I can only promise that if you read this book carefully, and follow my recommendations for only one week, you will finally understand why you have been unable to permanently lose weight in the past, and how you can assure that you will be successful in the future.

On the previous page, I cited John Milton's (1608-1674) claim in *Paradise Lost* that more people have died from an excessive ingestion of meat and drink than by all the other violent acts that have taken place on earth.[1] His pronouncement has been echoed by many others, as I will detail in the pages of this book, but such an assertion is misleading, for there is more to the damage of overeating than simply choosing what types of food to consume, and how much to eat and drink. It is true that gluttony can cause obesity, and the resultant gain in weight can lead to fatal complications, but anyone who compares the eating habits of overweight patients and their neighbors knows that some people can gain weight eating cucumber sandwiches for lunch, while others seem to nibble on cheese pizza all day long, and remain annoyingly slender for years. As one well-known physician summarized in the 1900s, one "subject burns, instantly and mercilessly, every stick of fuel delivered at his door, whether or not he needs the resulting hot fire roaring within, while the other, miser-like hoards the rest in vast piles, filling the house form cellar to garret."[2] There clearly is some type of relationship between a patient's weight and his or her "metabolism," yet no one has yet provided a satisfactory explanation for this frustrating disparity. If you have tried to convince your friends that you are not a "closet eater," but simply cannot seem to lose weight by consuming a moderate calorie intake, it is likely that they have politely accepted your excuse, and then turned away with a clear look of disbelief on their face, whispering to their friends that you don't get fat by eating a well-balanced diet.

Well, I am here to tell you that you can get fat by eating a well-balanced diet if you lack a substance in your blood that promotes the burning of fat stores, and I will show you how you can prove to your detractors that your problem with obesity is due to this genetic hormonal or enzymatic deficiency that is as yet undefined, but identifiable by a failure to quickly catabolize (break down) fat when you significantly reduce your calorie intake. You are similar to the overweight, fatigued patient who suffered from hypothyroidism before thyroid hormone was discovered in 1914 by the American biochemist Edward Kendall (1886-1972). You are like the tired, cachectic patient who suffered from uncontrolled Diabetes Mellitus until insulin was discovered in 1921 by the Canadian physicians Frederick Banting (1891-1941) and Charles Best (1899-1978). The reason you are fat, and many of your friends are not, is that they turn their fat stores into energy at low caloric intake levels, and you do not. The problem is no one has yet discovered the substance responsible for this condition.

Your particular ailment may be frustrating and dangerous in our modern era, but it was a definite advantage to your hunter-gatherer ancestors, who often went without food for long periods of time. The ability to maintain excess fat stores was life-saving back then, and may be the primary reason your particular descendants survived preferentially to the present day. The widespread availability of food in civilized countries today makes obesity an archaic defense mechanism, however, and puts your health at risk for a number of reasons, as I will explain shortly. Most medical doctors, and the majority of dieticians and other so-called experts, truly believe that your problem is one of over-eating, as is evident in the conclusion of Drs. MacCuish and Ford from the Royal Infirmary in Glasgow, Scotland, that the most important step in treating obesity is to "document the pattern of eating behaviour which has led to obesity, and to identify any obvious stresses which precipitate inappropriate eating."[3] While this approach may be suitable for some patients, it is not the answer for your genetic deficiency.

In the following pages, I am going to show you how you can find out if you have this hormonal or enzymatic defect, and what you can do to extend your life, so that when a medication is finally found to correct your deficiency, you will be able to reap the benefits. Trust me, with the economic incentives available for drug companies to discover this problem, an answer is on the horizon, and I do not think your children, who likely suffer from the same inherited defect, will have to fight the same battle of weight gain despite a relatively normal intake of calories. Along with a survival benefit by following my advice, you will save money by requiring less costly medications for Hypertension, Hypercholesterolemia, and Diabetes Mellitus, and you will be able to spend your savings on altering your clothes so they fit your more attractive physique. When Upton Sinclair (1878-1968), the prolific American author and Socialist, first became aware of the health benefits of fasting and weight loss, he noted how he had previously paid $15,000 to physicians and

2

druggists over the previous 6-8 years, and then had spent nothing in the year following the institution of his periodic water-fasts.[4] You, as well, will be able to save money on doctor bills and medications, and you will also be able to tell your friends that they were wrong to believe you were a closet-eater, unable to put forth the effort to follow a standard lo-cal diet. You must act now, however, for your obesity is not something you should passively accept, just because it is not easily cured.

II. A PRIMER ON THE DANGERS OF OBESITY

When I entered the private practice of medicine in 1972, the number one killer in America was heart disease, an illness caused by the blockage of small arteries to the heart and brain by cholesterol-containing plaques, a condition known as arteriosclerosis (atherosclerosis). In 2007, that statistic has changed very little. Despite the fact that great progress has been made in extending the age at which a fatal cardiovascular event takes place, people still primarily die because they have advanced arteriosclerosis. With all the fear generated today by the seemingly epidemic scourge of cancer, 652,486 Americans died of heart disease in 2004, while 553,091 succumbed to cancer.[5] Women die from a heart attack eight times more often than from breast cancer, even though the fear-factor of breast cancer gets most of the publicity.

These statistics are especially disconcerting in face of the advancements which have been made in the treatment of heart disease. Coronary Care Units (CCUs), which were developed for the first time in 1966 when I graduated medical school, have provided concentrated nursing care and cardiac monitoring to unstable patients, allowing them to timely receive medications which can treat the potentially fatal cardiac arrhythmias that accompany an acute myocardial infarction (MI). Coronary angiography, devised by Dr. Mason Sones (1919-1985) of the Cleveland Clinic in 1958, has provided cardiologists the means to prevent expansion of irreversible damage during a heart attack, by opening partially occluded coronary arteries so that a minimum of injury will take place. Those of us who were working on the frontline of medicine during that era of cardiac-care progress were exhilarated by the incredible improvement in the care of patients with myocardial infarctions and congestive heart failure, and we even believed that control of the disease was near-at-hand. But while the new techniques reduced the likelihood that you would immediately die from a heart attack by as much as 58%, they did not prevent the likelihood that another heart attack would occur in the near future, once again putting your life at risk. It is estimated that cardiac catheterization will be performed nearly 3 million times each year by the year 2010, saving countless of lives in the short-term, but the fact remains that the patient's underlying coronary artery disease will not be cured by this type of intervention alone.

To try and prevent heart attacks, rather than treat them once they have occurred, physicians have developed an extensive armamentarium of medications aimed at lowering serum cholesterol levels, a prime cause of the formation of arteriosclerotic plaques. Following the introduction of Mevacor (lovastatin) in 1987 by Merck, working with Sankyo Pharmaceutical in Japan, patients can now be offered a wide variety of cholesterol-lowering agents such as Statins (Zocor, Lipitor, Pravachol, Lescol, and Crestor), Fibrates (Lopid), Anion-exchange Resins (Questran, Colestid), Niacin, and Fish Oil supplements, just to mention a few. Newer products are being introduced each year, and it is estimated that pharmaceutical companies will take in over $30 billion yearly from this one class of drugs alone. While most studies do show some improvement in the recurrence rate of heart attack and stroke when patient's cholesterol levels are lowered by drug therapy, the results are not consistent, and the side-effects of the medications have become a major concern to both patients and physicians alike. Although lowering blood cholesterol levels by medication remains an important adjunct to the optimal care of patients with arteriosclerosis, it is not the panacea some cardiologists would have you believe, and weight control remains an important part of any total health program.

This overemphasis on the blood level of cholesterol alone brings me back to my earlier promise of being able to save your life in the opening sentence of this book. While the medical profession and the public have become enthralled with understanding and treating the deleterious effects of elevated blood cholesterol and coronary blockage, we have lost sight of the independent danger of obesity, an illness which causes arteriosclerosis to progress, even when the cholesterol level in the blood is normal.[6] As the average cholesterol level in the blood of patients worldwide continues to go down through the use of medication, the average weight of the population is going up at an alarming rate. Data from two National Health and Nutrition Examination Surveys (NHANES) in the United States has shown that the prevalence of obesity among adults aged 20-74 years increased from 15% in the 1976-1980 survey, to 32.9% in the 2003-2004 survey.[7] By 2008, the proportion of obese adults in the United States was 26.1%.[8] This dramatic doubling of the rate of obesity is not restricted to America, but is a worldwide problem, suggesting to some researchers that the increase might even be due to a virus epidemic.[9] Over one hundred million Americans, or three out of every five adults, now fit the category of being overweight or obese, while in Europe, about 20% of middle-aged people are obese, and a further 30% are overweight. According to the World Health Organization (WHO), obesity now affects more adults in the world than hunger.[10]

Obesity is dangerous because it is an independent risk factor for many serious disease states, including Diabetes Mellitus, Dyslipidemia, Osteoarthritis, Sleep Apnea, Gout, Gallstones, Fatty Liver Disease, Venous Thromboembolism, and Hypertension, in addition to Arteriosclerosis. It also is associated with an increased rate of developing cancers of the ovary, endometrium, breast, gallbladder, colon, prostate, esophagus, thyroid, and gallbladder.[11] Through these epidemiologic relationships, it is estimated that obesity is responsible for over 280,000 deaths each year in the United States alone,[12] and that the overall increase in mortality is about 15% for every 10% a person is above the normal weight.[13]

Obesity not only leads to fatal medical problems, it also creates excess pain and suffering by worsening various chronic inflammatory conditions through the excess production of adipokine hormones, such as TNF-alpha (tumor necrosis factor alpha) and IL-6 (interleukin-6), which set off the body's inflammatory response. It increases the incidence of reproductive problems in women, including menstrual irregularities and infertility, and causes excessive wear and tear on tendons and joints, leading to painful back and lower extremity disorders. These chronic complaints cost our health-care system a great deal of money, accounting for almost 5.5% of our annual national medical expense, reaching estimates as high as $40 billion a year. This total does not include other expenses, such as loss of productivity from sick leave, and higher insurance premiums and disability, which can add up to as much as $122.9 billion a year in the United States alone.[14] This is an enormous financial burden, given the fact that cancer treatment in the United States in 2004 was estimated to have cost $72.1 billion.[15]

How can obesity increase all of these seemingly unrelated problems, simply through the accumulation of excessive weight? The answer is not simple, but one critical mechanism is the development of "insulin resistance," a condition first uncovered in 1936 by Sir Harold Percival Himsworth (1905-1993) of the University College Hospital Medical Center in London, and named Syndrome X by Dr. Gerald Reaven from Stanford University in 1988. Insulin, the only hormone in the body capable of lowering blood glucose levels, is produced by the specialized beta-cells of the Islets of Langerhans in the pancreas. Under conditions of normal metabolism, insulin is released in response to the ingestion of food, directing the insulin-sensitive tissues of the body to absorb glucose. The pancreas of patients with juvenile type I Diabetes Mellitus does not produce insulin, and as a result their glucose levels are greatly elevated, eventually leading to death if the patient is not given insulin injections. In an "insulin resistance" patient, an insulin response to the ingestion of food does take place, but it is diminished and delayed, resulting in a continued elevation of blood sugar levels. This stimulates the pancreas to release more insulin, eventually leading to hyperinsulinemia (elevated insulin levels in the blood). Because the insulin release is delayed, it takes place when the sugar in the blood has finally begun to decrease, resulting in hypoglycemia (low blood sugar), which increases hunger and – you guessed it – an increased intake of food and further elevations of blood sugar. The cycle, in essence, feeds upon itself (no pun intended), and because insulin promotes the formation of fat cells throughout the body, the excessive amounts of insulin in the blood results in significant weight gain, a reaction which also occurs in diabetic patients who begin insulin therapy for the first time. I will discuss this issue of insulin resistance, which is also a hallmark of type II Diabetes Mellitus, in many other sections of this book, but it is important for you to realize at the very outset that many of these problems are controllable if you can lose weight and learn to eat less food, at least until medication becomes available to attack this problem by correction of your hormonal deficiency.

Although it generally is obvious from mere visual inspection alone whether a person is overweight, the diagnosis of obesity in medical studies is often determined by measuring the body mass index (BMI), a statistical measure invented by the Belgian polymath Adolphe Quetelet (1796-1874) in the nineteenth century C.E. This calculation is made by either dividing the weight of the patient in kilograms (2.2 lbs = 1 kg) by the square of the height in meters (1 in = 0.0254 m), or by dividing the weight in pounds by the square of the height in inches, and then multiplying by 703. Values from 18.5-24.9 are considered optimal, 25-29.9 is overweight, 30-34.9 is obese, and over 35 is morbidly obese. Very few individuals actually fall within the optimal category, and being mildly overweight on the BMI scale is not a significant risk for the development of heart attack or stroke. If your BMI is 30 or above, however, you are definitely in the class of person who should follow *KetoFast*, since a BMI between 30-40 is a "moderate risk" for developing medical complications, and above 40 is a "high risk."[16] There are many tomograms available on the worldwide web which allow you to input your own height and weight and immediately know your BMI number without testing your mathematical skills, but it is not necessary to resort to this calculation while you follow the *KetoFast* diet, since the change in your weight will clearly reflect your success or failure.

If you don't have access to a BMI calculator, or if you could care less about how scientifically fat you are, you can still easily tell if your weight puts you at an increased health risk by simply measuring your waist circumference at your umbilicus (bellybutton). A total of more than 35 inches (88 cm) in women, and more than 40 inches (102 cm) in men, is indicative of a higher health risk than those with lower levels. If your waist size is below these numbers, feel free to read this book for educational reasons, but your concern should be toward maintenance of a healthy weight by proper exercise and dietary control. Don't get too cocky, however, for even if you are not one of those who are genetically prone to obesity, you can still become at risk for health hazards by gaining weight through poor eating habits.

III. WHY YOU ARE OBESE AND WHAT YOU CAN DO TO LOSE WEIGHT

As I discussed in the Introduction to this book, if you are overweight, and have failed multiple attempts at losing weight with moderate calorie restriction, you likely have a genetic defect that is not yet clearly defined. That the problem is genetic is consistent with the fact that obesity, like Diabetes Mellitus and Hypercholesterolemia, often runs in families. If both of your parents are obese, there is a 70% chance that you will become obese as well, while if your parents are of normal weight, there is only an 8% chance you will become obese.[17] That this is not due to similar eating habits alone is attested to by the fact that identical twins who are raised apart develop a body habitus which resembles that of their biologic parents and siblings, more than it does their adoptive parents, indicating that the problem is one of "nature," and not "nurture."[18]

Animal research has supported this assessment by uncovering genetic defects in mice which lead to excessive weight gain. The most well-studied of these systems is the Ob gene, first discovered in 1994 by Jeffrey Friedman and his colleagues at Rockefeller University. In homozygous ob/ob mice, the genetic mutation results in a condition that includes increased food intake, reduced energy expenditure, and elevated insulin levels, leading to massive obesity and non-insulin dependent Diabetes Mellitus, a syndrome similar to what is seen in human beings. The underlying cause is a defect in a gene which encodes the peptide hormone leptin, a substance produced by adipocytes (fat cells) and secreted into the blood. Leptin operates as an important regulator of the mass of adipose tissue in the body, inhibiting food intake and stimulating energy expenditure. When the gene is mutated, an inactive leptin protein is produced, or in some cases no protein at all, and this results in a loss of appetite suppression. When leptin is administered to these animals, the multiple metabolic disturbances are corrected, and the weight of the animal returns to normal.

The possibility that leptin may play a similar role in some cases of human obesity has recently been supported by the finding that certain families also appear to have a defective leptin gene that causes them to become obese. First discovered by a team at the Cambridge Institute for Medical Research in 1998, two very obese children from a highly consanguineous family were found to have low levels of leptin in their blood, an indication that they had a mutation in the leptin gene. The researchers treated one of the children with leptin injections made by the drug company Amgen, and within two weeks the child's appetite returned to normal, followed by a sustained, dramatic weight loss.[19] Since then, 12 more subjects have been treated by the Cambridge group

9

with recombinant human leptin, and all have shown improvement in their clinical weight abnormalities.[20]   Similar results have been reported by researchers at the University of California in adults from other families.[21]

Commercial methods to measure leptin levels are not yet available, and even if they were, it is likely that the leptin injections that are able to be used in research studies are years away from approval by the Federal Drug Administration (FD) for general use. There are a myriad of other hormones, in addition to leptin, which have been found to control appetite and lead to excessive weight gain, however, and these may prove to be even more effective in the future. One such compound is ghrelin, a compound produced by P/D1 cells lining the stomach, which acts to counteract the effects of leptin. Discovered in 1999 as a stimulator of the secretion of growth hormone from the anterior pituitary gland, ghrelin is controlled by the same gene which encodes the production of obestatin, a ghrelin-associated peptide found in 2005 by researchers at Stanford University School of Medicine which decreases appetite. Gherlin levels increase before meals, adding to your feelings of hunger, and then decrease after meals, helping to lead to satiety, the exact opposite of what is seen with leptin. Blood levels of gherlin only decrease following the ingestion of food or glucose, and not water, suggesting that gastric distension is not a factor in this equation. In rodents, administration of ghrelin, either centrally or peripherally, increases food intake and body weight, and in humans given ghrelin intravenously, there is a potent increase in food intake of 28%.[22] It has been found that lack of sleep increases ghrelin levels in the blood, possibly explaining why short sleep duration may also increase the incidence of obesity. One interesting sidelight of ghrelin is that patients who have lost weight by dietary methods have been found to have elevated ghrelin levels, while patients who have undergone gastric-bypass (bariatric) surgery have showed lowered ghrelin levels.[23] This may explain why there is less of an appetite stimulus following the surgical technique, compared to dieting alone.

If you have carefully read my book up to this point, however, you will realize that I do not feel that these genetic abnormalities are the cause of your obesity, since your problem is not one of gluttony, but of the inability to lose weight at relatively moderate levels of calorie intake. In my experience, this is true of many overweight individuals, and is the reason why almost all patients will lose some weight when they rigidly stick to a low-calorie diet, but then regain it when they return to a more normal intake. While substances like leptin and gherlin are advancing our understanding of obesity due to pathologic acceleration of hunger, there must be other pathways that lead to abnormal weight gain.

One compound which may help explain your particular problem is adiponectin, a hormone secreted by adipocytes which sensitizes the body to insulin. Lower adiponectin concentrations in humans has been associated with greater visceral obesity, insulin resistance, and incidence of type 2 Diabetes Mellitus in certain populations. In mice, treatment with adiponectin can reduce body-weight gain, increase insulin sensitivity, and decrease lipid levels, but human studies have not yet been conducted. If you lack adiponectin, or a substance like it, or if your enzymatic pathway which is the substrate for adiponectin is abnormal, you will gain weight at levels of calorie intake that other people will not. Once again, a test to measure the level of adiponectin in your blood is not commercially available. Although there is no evidence yet that modification of adiponectin levels will help you lose weight, some dietary advocates have promoted the ingestion of anthocyanins, pigments found in fruits with deep red, blue and purple colors, which are known to increase the production of adiponectin.[24] I have no problem with your taking these fruits as part of your menu choices on the *KetoFast* diet, but be sure to measure the calorie content carefully, since fruits are relatively calorie-dense.

There are likely many other substances which affect the formation and catabolism of adipose tissue, and deficiency of one of these compounds may explain why many patients who are obese tend to store fat more easily than their leaner counterparts. This tendency for some patients to easily gain weight has been recognized for many years, as evidenced by the conclusion of Drs. Otto Folin & Willey Glover Denis, from Massachusetts General Hospital in Boston in 1915 that obese patients "probably tend to utilize it [fat] less readily," then patients who are thin.[25] I first became aware of this abnormality many years ago, when one of my patients had to undergo elective surgery for gallstones, and the surgeon would not operate until she lost some of her excess weight. She was morbidly obese, carrying most of her weight in her abdominal wall, which put her at a significant increased risk of complications from the surgery, since this was the era when a long abdominal incision was necessary, rather than the limited techniques utilized today by laproscopic surgical techniques. Because time was of the essence, and the patient had failed many prior attempts at dieting in the past, I admitted her to a hospital to initiate a zero-calorie water-fast, which I had utilized on other patients when rapid weight loss was necessary. This was in the days before health maintenance organizations (HMOs), when doctors could do anything they believed was in the patient's best interest, even if it was not cost-effective. It also was before acceptance of severe calorie restriction or zero-calorie diets, so hospitalization was a necessary precaution to assure the patient was carefully monitored during the starvation phase. The regimen consisted of no food at all, with *ad libitum* intake of water and supplementation of micronutrient minerals and vitamins.

Before you cringe with the thought of not eating any food at all for more than a few hours, let me point out that fasting for days or weeks at a time has been utilized for over 5,000 years, not simply to lose weight, but because of the health and spiritual benefits that accrue from living on water alone. The ancient Greeks utilized fasts, as did the ancient Chinese and Indian civilizations. The Jewish faithful fast on Yom Kippur (Day of Atonement) and six other days during the year, highlighting the fact that both Moses and Elijah were said to have fasted for 40 days before their communions with God.[26] Catholics fast during Lent, on Ash Wednesday and Good Friday, following the lead of Jesus Christ, who fasted for 40 days in the wilderness after his baptism.[27] The Eastern Orthodox Church is more zealous than the Catholic Church in this regard, recommending as many as 180 days for fasting in the course of a year. Hindus fast on New Moon days, Ekadasi, and during various festivals; the Baha'i fast from sunrise to sunset during the month of Ala; and Buddhists fast on full-moon days and certain holidays. In Islam, fasting is the third of five pillars of religious obligation, and over one billion Muslims throughout the world fast between sunrise and sunset during the month of Ramadan.[28] Most Anglican and mainline Protestant churches leave the question of fasting to the individual member, but important fast-days are recommended in the Book of Common Prayer. That more than spiritual benefit accrues to those who practice fasting is evident from the fact that Mormons, who generally fast one day a month, have a lower rate of coronary artery disease than the general population.[29]

When I admitted my patient to the hospital for a prolonged weight-loss fast, I did not consider these religious benefits, but only encouraged her to follow my recommendations in order to prepare her for surgery as soon as possible. She had no problem adhering to the fast, and stated that there were almost no pangs of hunger after the first day. I now know that this is a well-known reaction among fast-enthusiasts, but at the time I did not realize how much hunger had to do with the sight, smell, and expectation of food. Most people who go on water-fasts frequently say that it is easier to eat nothing at all, than to try and eat a small amount. As Ivan Pavlov (1849-1946), the Russian physiologist and physician, proved in experiments on dogs, the sight and smell of food is a powerful stimulant to the production of gastric juices, and when you physically do not eat at all, this outpouring of digestive desire is suppressed. In addition, when you know that food is going to be entirely withheld, your hunger is not as potent.

In order to determine when my patient actually began to turn to her fat stores as an energy source, I assayed her urine for ketones four times a day. This technique takes advantage of the fact that during fat catabolism, large fatty acids are broken into smaller molecules, known as ketone bodies (acetoacetic acid, beta-hydroxybutyric acid, and acetone). These ketone bodies build up in the blood, and when the levels increase above 0.1-0.2 mM/ml, they become detectable in the urine. During prolonged fasting, the amount can increase 70-fold, reaching levels of 10-12 mM/ml. This degree of ketone elevation in the blood and urine is not as dangerous as diabetic ketoacidosis (DKA), a potentially fatal complication of uncontrolled Diabetes Mellitus, where ketone levels can reach 20-40 mM/ml. In DKA, the pH of the blood falls below 3.5 (normal 3.5-4.5), leading to widespread tissue necrosis and functional deficits. In starvation ketosis, however, the pH remains normal. One benefit of elevated ketones without acidosis (ketosis) is an associated suppression of appetite. In addition to a suppression of appetite by the absence of the sight and smell of food, the elevation of ketones in the blood makes you less desirous of food. More importantly, by measuring the excretion of ketones into the urine, you can determine exactly when you are actually burning the fat in your body, thereby allowing you to manage your own metabolic pathway without elaborate medical testing. If you spill ketones in your urine without eating, you are burning fat. If you are fasting, but do not spill ketones in your urine, you are in a hibernation-mode, where fat stores are being preserved rather than being converted into an energy source. While this is good if you are a bear sleeping away a long cold winter's night, it is bad if you are attempting to lose weight.

The test for ketones in the urine is very easy, and only requires dipping a coated reagent strip (Ketostix) into urine collected in a cup, or simply passing the strip through the urinary stream as you urinate. You then wait for 10-15 seconds, and compare the color of the strip to a color chart which tells you if you have negative, trace, small, moderate, or large amounts of ketones in the urine. The strip is capable of detecting 5 mg/dl of acetoacetate, but is not reactive to acetone. By measuring the level of ketones in the urine four times each day, you can control the development of ketosis in your body quite safely, as long as you are not a medication-dependent diabetic.

To my amazement, the woman did not show any sign of ketones in the urine for three days, despite the intake of zero calories under controlled conditions. Most normal-weight patients will begin to show ketones in the urine when they are on a twelve to twenty-four hour fast before having their bloods drawn for a routine History and Physical examination, although some individuals may take up to 24-36 hours. This ability to burn fat as an energy source early in the fasting process allows most people to control their weight by simple dietary methods alone. If they gain too much weight, they simply lower their calorie intake for a few days, begin to burn their fat into ketones, and weight reduction takes place quite readily. But this woman, as I was subsequently to find with every other obese patient I treated with a zero-calorie diet in my practice, did not begin to burn her fat for over three days, preventing her from quickly and easily losing weight by sensible dietary restrictions. Moreover, when she began to eat food, her ketone production in the urine

13

ceased after she began to eat 600 calories per day. **600 calories per day!!** Can you imagine how discouraging it was to both of us when we found that her weight loss would stop for prolonged periods of time when she ate more than 600 calories a day?

At the time, I thought her condition may have been relatively unique, but as I will discuss shortly, it is now known that many patients must conform to a very-low-calorie diet (VLCD), which provides only 300-600 calories/day, in order to lose weight. I also eventually learned that my patient was not the first of her kind, for the patient that Folin & Denis described in 1915 was also an obese woman who had to undergo a water-fast in order to prepare for surgery of a large ventral abdominal wall hernia. They concluded that their technique of utilizing successive moderate periods of starvation constitutes "a perfectly safe, harmless, and effective method for reducing the weight of those suffering from obesity."[30] It took almost a century for most of the medical profession to understand the meaning of their finding, and for you to finally realize the importance of this plan in explaining the reasons for your overweight condition.

Why did this patient, and so many like her, take three days of starvation to begin to burn their fat cells, and then turn fat catabolism off when they ingested 600 calories a day? The answer is not apparent if you do a literature search on the subject, but I believe that the explanation lies in the fact that there is some defect or deficiency of a substance, most likely a hormone or enzymatic pathway, that directs the catabolism of fat during periods of food deprivation. From an evolutionary standpoint, this defect would have been an advantage during eras when drought and climactic conditions severely limited the supply of food. Families who inherited this condition could sustain life for longer periods of time by mimicking the conditions which characterize hibernating bears. Today, however, such a benefit is not useful, and in order to turn lemon into lemonade, you are going to have to grin and bear your unique nature, and find comfort in the fact that your ancestors profited for a few hundred thousand years so that you could now read this book and try and control your weight through the technique of *KetoFast*.

What the *KetoFast* diet does is to take advantage of this ketone excretion and provide you with a means by which you can tell if you are in a satisfactory negative caloric mode to cause weight loss. It shows you when your adipose tissue is being converted into energy so that you can be assured of losing weight with the amount of calories you are eating. If you follow the precepts outlined in the pages which follow, I guarantee you will lose weight and then be able to maintain your desired weight level by testing the ability of your body to continue to burn fat cells. Despite the fact that many modern dietary gurus tell you that calories are not the problem, and that it is the type of food you eat, rather than the total calories consumed, it is my opinion that you should forget all that pedantic nonsense and pay attention to one major truism: **Calories are the cornerstone of weight reduction.** There is no reliable evidence that calorie for calorie, any food substance will lead to greater weight loss than another over an extended period of time, although there are some claims that eating vegetables alone will allow one to gain less weight than eating a similar calorie intake from animal-based foods because of thermogenesis. In my opinion, a calorie is a calorie, and it does not matter if it came from protein, carbohydrate, or fat.

Although many patients will lose weight if they can limit their caloric intake to a low enough level, even a 100-calorie excess above this threshold level can slow, or even stop, weight loss. This means you must accurately measure your calorie intake if you are going to maintain a proper VLCD that is not artificially prepared. To assist you in managing this sharp restriction, all of the recipes contained within this book are 100-calories or less, within 10%. You can therefore design your own diet, remaining within 100-calorie increments to fine-tune your total intake, and eat healthy foods, naturally prepared, rather than products that are composed of powders from a variety of predigested provisions. It may seem incredulous at first, but you can eat small portions of foods of your own choosing, and by checking the excretion of ketones in your urine, you can accurately determine how many calories you can eat in order to effectively lose weight.

IV. UNDERSTANDING FAT CATABOLISM

OK, you now know why I believe you are obese, and why you have failed many diet plans in the past.   You also know how you can tell if you fit this mode by undergoing a zero-calorie fast, and test your urine four times a day to see when you spill ketones.   If it takes up to 2 days or more, you are in the club. The longer it takes for you to begin utilizing your fat stores, the more severe your problem.   I now want to give you a short physiology lesson to explain why it is necessary for you to carefully follow the calorie restrictions I am going to outline in this book, in order to catabolize fat cells in your body and lose weight.

Adipose tissue consists primarily of triglycerides, which are fatty acids combined with a carrier glycerol molecule.   Every cell in the body needs fatty acids for proper function and reproduction, but in most organs, fatty acids are only a minor component of the cell structure.   In fat cells, however, triglycerides make up more than 95% of the cell space.   Although the fatty acids released from the triglycerides during the catabolic process are capable of producing energy, the body does not begin to utilize them until the supply of glucose from exogenous and endogenous sources is thoroughly depleted. Mammalian organisms primarily rely on glucose, a sugar compound composed of carbon, hydrogen, and oxygen, to provide their energy needs. Glucose, from the Greek word for "sweet," is present at the cellular level as a monosaccharide, the smallest molecular structure of sugar.   In addition to glucose, monosaccharides also exist as fructose (fruit sugar), galactose (milk sugar), and ribose (a component of DNA).   Two monosaccharides can be combined into a disaccharide, which is the primary component for glucose in food, including sucrose (glucose-fructose), which is ordinary table sugar; lactose (galactose-glucose), which is the sugar found in milk products; and the stereoisomers maltose (glucose-glucose in the 1-4 *a* linkage), which is found in malt products and cereals, trehalose (glucose-glucose in the 1,1-glucoside *a* bond), and cellobiose (glucose-glucose in the 1-4 *b* linkage). Disaccharides can also be joined together by multiple glycosidic linkages to form large polysaccharides, such as starch, cellulose, glycogen, and chitin. Potato, rice, wheat, and maize are the major sources of starch in the human diet, and cellulose, which provides much of the fiber content of the food we eat, is the structural component of plants.   Glycogen is the storage form for glucose, concentrated primarily in the liver, kidney, and muscular tissue.

Disaccharides and polysaccharides are broken down into monosaccharides during the digestive process, and then absorbed into the blood.   If not immediately utilized as an energy source, the excess glucose molecules are converted into glycogen for storage. When you go on a water-

17

fast, and restrict the intake of glucose from carbohydrate ingestion, the body immediately turns to the catabolism of glycogen to provide a continuing source of glucose. Our glycogen stores are limited, however, because it is not an efficient form of energy storage for long-term use. Each gram of glycogen provides 4 calories of available energy, but to store 1 gram of glycogen, you also have to accumulate 1-2 grams of intracellular water, so that the total weight of the particle is a significant load as an energy reserve. Our body therefore only stores enough glycogen molecules to supply the necessary quantities of glucose for about twelve hours of fasting. The average-sized man will contain approximately 350 gms of glycogen, providing about 1200-1500 calories.[31]

Once the glycogen stores are depleted, the body then turns to protein catabolism to provide glucose through the process of gluconeogenesis. That is why normal individuals begin to spill ketones after a 12-24 hour fast; they have to first utilize their available glycogen stores. The first response to occur is that protein is broken down into carbon atoms, which then are reformulated into the glucose molecule.[32] Protein, however, is a vital component of normal bodily function, providing the structure of skeletal muscles locomotion and power, and smooth muscles for cardiac and digestive function. If too much protein is lost in order to provide energy needs, the resultant deficiency would prove detrimental to our health. In addition, protein requires an even greater aqueous environment than glycogen, with the weight of muscular tissue containing only 20% of the weight in actual protein molecules. Our body has therefore evolved a superior method of energy storage in the form of fat, and the catabolism of protein is short-lived as fat stores begin to be converted to glucose.

Fat is stored in an extra-aqueous environment, with 1 gram of adipose tissue having less than 10% water content, providing almost 9.4 calories of available energy per gram of tissue, rather than the 4 calories available from carbohydrates and protein. The average man will store about 140,000 calories as fat, 24,000 calories as protein, and 1200 calories as glycogen,[33] and obese patients can contain as many as 300,000 calories in their expansive fat stores. In order to lose large amounts of weight, you must force your body to catabolize fat as an energy source, but this means that you must first deplete your internal stores of glycogen, and then initiate a short period of gluconeogenesis before beginning the process of fat catabolism. This process takes time, especially in patients who are obese from a genetic deficiency of their catabolic process.

To understand why you seem to gain weight much more rapidly than you lose it, you have to understand how our bodies regulate the equilibrium between anabolic activity, which puts weight on, and catabolic activity, which takes weight off. We all require a constant supply of energy to maintain life, even when we are completely at rest. Any kind of activity will increase our energy needs, even when we eat, since energy is used up in the digestive process. The rise in the metabolic rate after eating is known as the "thermic effect of food" (TEF), and with a mixed diet, about 6-10% of the metabolizable energy ingested can be lost as heat. About 75% of this response is due to the energy cost of digestion, absorption, metabolism, and storage of foodstuffs, while the remainder is believed to be due to activation of the sympathetic nervous system. The thermogenic effect of protein is the greatest, followed by carbohydrate and then fat. It is estimated that as much as 30% of the protein calorie total is dissipated by the digestive process, while with fat this amount drops to only 2-3%.

The minimum amount of energy required for the sedentary maintenance of life, in the post-absorptive state when the digestive system is inactive and the body is at rest, is known as the basal metabolic rate (BMR), or resting metabolic rate (RMR). When you go on a water-fast, or a VLCD, the body senses the deprivation of ingested calories and attempts to reduce energy outflow by reducing the BMR an average of 15-21%.[34] This adaptive mechanism has evolved to protect ourselves from significant rapid weight loss during periods of starvation, and can amount to as much as 40-50% of our usual energy requirements. In most people, the BMR amounts to about 1000 calories per m2 body surface area per day, and since the average person measures between 1.5-2.0 m2 body surface area, 1500-2000 calories must be provided each day to maintain normal body weight under relatively quiescent living conditions. The brain utilizes about 400 calories of this energy requirement, the viscera 1000 calories, and the muscle 600 calories, depending on the extent of exercise.[35]

Many physicians have pointed to this reduction in BMR as a negative effect of utilizing fasting or VLCDs as an aid to weight loss, positing that the lowered metabolic rate reduces your likelihood of weight loss. Although based on factual physiologic data, such a conclusion fails to realize that significant weight loss does not require you to maintain your normal BMR, but rather to force your body to utilize fat cells as a source of energy, rather than glycogen and muscles. Effective weight loss does not begin until the glycogen stores are used up, and fat begins to be converted into ketone bodies as an energy source. Until you redirect fat catabolism to energy production, you will not continue to lose significant amounts of adipose tissue. A lowered BMR that utilizes fat as an energy source is better for weight loss, than a higher BMR that is burning the food you eat. In addition, the initial lowering of the BMR is not a permanent effect, and can return to normal levels with time and exercise.

Just because you are burning fat as an energy source does not mean that your weight will drop precipitately, however, since you have about 30-40 billion fat cells in your body, and each one can expand to hundreds of times its initial size. It is obvious that this modification will take some effort to finally normalize your weight problem. Each fat cell is composed of about 95% triglycerides, with small amounts of free fatty acids (primarily myristic, palmitic, palmitoleic, stearic, oleic, and linoleic acid), diglyceride, cholesterol, and phospholipid. The fat cells are distributed differently in men and women, with the android pattern in men characterized by fat distribution primarily in the upper body above the waist, the so-called "apple" appearance, while the gynecoid pattern in women disperses most of the fat in the lower body, including the lower abdomen, buttocks, hips and thighs, the so-called "pear" shape. Although women are often distressed by their particular fat pattern, they have a better prognosis of not developing heart attacks than men, since the male pattern of visceral obesity is a key determinant of insulin resistance.[36] Recent data from Germany suggests that this increased risk of arteriosclerosis from visceral obesity is particularly evident in patients with ectopic fat accumulation in the liver, as measured by magnetic resonance imaging (MRI).[37]

When the body finally turns to fat stores as an energy source, triglycerides are first broken down into fatty acids and glycerol by a hormone-sensitive lipase, an enzyme which is activated by the hormones epinephrine (adrenalin) and glucagon, and inhibited by insulin. Epinephrine, also known as the "fight or flight" hormone, is secreted by the adrenal glands, while glucagon is secreted by the alpha cells of the pancreas in response to a protein meal. The fatty acids are then catabolized in stages by a series of four reactions which take place in the mitochondria of cells, each of which removes an acetyl-coenzyme A molecule by a different acyl dehydrogenase enzyme. One of these enzymes, known as medium chain acyl-coenzyme A dehydrogenase (MCAD), is deficient in children with an autosomal recessive disorder that generally shows up in the first few years of life, and is one of the rarer causes of sudden infant death syndrome (SIDS). These unfortunate infants develop profound hypoglycemia during fasting, due to their inability to initiate the beta-oxidation cycle of fatty acid catabolism.[38] The parents of these children have been shown to be asymptomatic carriers of the defective gene, with intermediate levels of activity of the MCAD enzyme, and it is possible that a similar type of genetic deficiency, of milder nature, could explain why you do not easily convert your adipose tissue to glucose during calorie deprivation.[39] Children with MCAD never show ketones in their urine when they are deprived of feeding, an indication that they are totally unable to convert triglycerides into fatty acids. Similar deficiency states have been described for very long-chain acyl-coenzyme A dehydrogenase deficiency (VLCAD), and short-chain acyl-coenzyme A dehydrogenase deficiency (SCAD). The detection of these enzymes is not readily available in commercial laboratories, and there is no treatment for those with the full-blown disease except for dietary supplements, which bypass the necessity of breaking down triglycerides into their fatty acids components. It is possible, however, that future studies may make this defect a possible treatable condition, both for those with the total enzymatic deficiency, and even for obese patients who may have a partial deficiency.

Another inherited disease which interferes with the catabolism of fatty acids is carnitine palmitoyltransferase II (CPT2) deficiency, a generally fatal condition when it presents in infants between the ages of 6 and 24 months. Adults, however, can present with a milder myopathic form of the disease, which is characterized by recurrent episodes of muscle pain (myalgia) and weakness, and intermittent dark-colored urine due to the excessive excretion of myoglobin. These patients are often misdiagnosed as having heart attacks during their episodes of chest pain because of elevated levels of muscle enzymes in their blood. Because fatty acids cannot be converted into energy when glycogen stores are diminished, excess long-chain fatty acids build up in the tissues, and muscles are catabolized as an energy source, leading to muscle pain from rhabdomyolysis triggered by prolonged exercise or fasting.[40] During starvation, ketonuria fails to appear, but the clinical presentation of severe muscle pain overshadows any confusion which may arise in obese patients described in this book. As with the MCAD deficiency, however, it is possible that some obese patients may have learned to refrain from allowing their body to turn to fatty acids as an energy source because of recurrent muscle pain.

It is important to realize that these fatty acid components of triglycerides are not related to the fatty acids which are well-known to most educated consumers today because of the publicity surrounding the dangers of dietary saturated fatty acids. Although this issue has more to do with affiliated health risks of arteriosclerosis than weight gain or loss, I think it is important for you to understand why the recipes in this book are designed to satisfy concerns of each of these serious health problems, so I am going to summarize some of the physiology and terminology of dietary fatty acids to enable you to make an informed decision about what foods and supplements to choose as you learn to decrease your total daily food intake in order to burn fatty acids as an energy source.

If all of the valence bonds of the carbon atom in a fatty acid are filled with hydrogen atoms, the compound is termed a saturated fatty acid (SFA), while if there are some open bonds present, it is labeled as an unsaturated fatty acid (UFA). Unsaturated fatty acids are considered healthier because they have a lesser chance of promoting the development of arteriosclerosis. If the fatty acid has one double bond between two carbon molecules, it is termed a monounsaturated fat (MUFA), while if there two or more double bonds on the same side of the chain (cis), it is called polyunsaturated (PUFA). The only two

PUFAs which the body cannot synthesize de-novo are linoleic acid and linolenic acid, the so-called "essential fatty acids." These substances must be ingested in either the food we eat, or by supplements available over-the-counter (OTC).

All fats and oils we consume are composed of a combination of these fatty acids, with beef fat comprised of 51% SFA, 44% MUFA, and 4% PUFA; butter 54% SFA, 30% MUFA, and 4% PUFA; margarine 18% SFA, 48% MUFA, and 29% PUFA; olive oil 14% SFA, 77% MUFA, and 9% PUFA; and safflower oil 9% SFA, 12% MUFA, and 78% PUFA.[41] Since polyunsaturated fats are believed to be much healthier by today's standards, safflower oil is often preferred as a dietary oil supplement, given its high PUFA content. Safflower and flaxseed oils oxidize the most rapidly when heated, however, so it is more common to find olive oil in recipes that require cooking, because it is low in SFAs. Extra-virgin olive oil is often used because it is generally believed to have a superior taste, rather than a healthier composition.

While naturally-occurring fatty acids are composed primarily of these compounds, during the chemical extraction to make artificial oils, hydrogenated unsaturated fats can transform into trans-fatty acids (TFAs) by adding hydrogen atoms to different sides of the carbon chain then occurs naturally, hence the "trans" nomenclature, rather than the more normal "cis" configuration. This industrial process was first developed in the early 1900s by hydrogenating cottonseed oil into a product called "Crisco" by Proctor & Gamble, and it rapidly was accepted as an alternative to the use of butter, margarine and animal fats in the cooking process because it was cheap and remained stable at room temperature, eliminating the need for refrigeration. Fast-food companies quickly began to include these products in their food processing, but it was not long before evidence that the ingestion of TFAs increased the risk of coronary artery disease began to appear in the medical literature.[42] By 1994, the consumption of trans-fats was postulated to have caused 30,000 deaths annually in the United States from heart disease alone.[43] The resultant clamor against the use of TFAs rose to such a pitch that the process of formulating Crisco was modified to eliminate TFAs in January 2007.[44] These by-products are still widespread in packaged and fast-foods, however, and you should be diligent in your reading of labels to avoid foods which contain partially-hydrogenated vegetable oils, hydrogenated vegetable oils, or shortening, as well as those where the values of the unsaturated, polyunsaturated, and monounsaturated fats add up to less than the total fats, an indication that TFAs are present.

I want to point out that while polyunsaturated fats are preferable to monounsaturated fats as a principle of general health, and while TFAs acids are an artificial and unhealthy substitute to natural oils, the caloric contributions of the various fatty acids are the same, and if you are dieting to lose weight, it is not more beneficial to eat polyunsaturated fats, simply because they are healthier than their monounsaturated cousins, if it means increasing your caloric intake in the process. For *KetoFast* purposes, it is the total calorie count that matters, and not the food content. While I recommend extra-virgin olive oil in most of the recipes of this book, you can choose any type of cooking oil you want, as long as you keep the total intake of calories down to the recommended levels.

Once catabolism of fat begins, and the triglycerides are broken down into their individual fatty acid molecules, the fatty acids are then oxidized into acetyl groups in the liver or kidneys, and diffused into the blood as acetoacetic acid or hydroxybutyrate. These ketone bodies are then carried to other tissues throughout the body, where they provide the primary source of energy during periods of glucose lack. The primary ketone body excreted into the urine is hydroxybutyrate, with acetone and acetoacetic acid accounting for less than 20% of the total ketone output. Acetoacetic acid is slowly changed to acetone, which is expired in the breath, as well as being excreted into the urine, causing the bad breath odor often found during zero-calorie fasts. Mouthwash or breath mints may become a necessary adjunct during Stage I and II, but the problem is only temporary, and a small price to pay for the successful loss of weight which takes place once you begin to burn your fat away. If the problem is not corrected by these simple maneuvers, you can drink mint tea, which contains chlorophyll, to help neutralize the offensive odor of halitosis.

Dr. Robert Atkins (1930-2003) has promoted this production of ketones in his high-fat, low-carbohydrate diet, which was first introduced in 1972, and updated in 1992. Atkins uses animal products to make up 90% of the calories in his diet, 60-75% coming from fat. Not only does ketosis develop when you utilize your own fat stores as an energy source, it also develops when you ingest large amounts of fat, leading to a state which Atkins labels as "Benign Dietary Ketosis (BDK)," his "secret weapon of supereffective dieting."[45] In essence, what Atkins attempts to do is to deplete your glycogen stores by removing carbohydrates from your diet, and then forcing energy to be derived from the high fat content of both your endogenous fat stores, and the large amounts of fat ingested on a daily basis. Ketosis in the Atkins diet is primarily derived from the utilization of the fat in your food, however, rather than from your internal stores of fat alone, and the presence of ketones in the urine does not assure you that you are catabolizing your adipose tissue, although some degree of weight loss is common. Because ketosis is associated with a reduced appetite, you are less hungry on the Atkins diet than on equivalent calorie intakes from high protein or carbohydrate plans. In my opinion, however, the excessive ingestion of a high-fat diet is not healthy, both because it accentuates your taste for foods which are universally felt to be atherogenic and carcinogenic, and because it does not allow you to rely on the ketone test in your urine to assure you are burning your own body fat. In addition, although many people will lose weight by following this diet, the amount of weight actually lost is not great, averaging only about 10 pounds at the end of one year.[46] I therefore do not suggest you attempt to eat a high-fat content once you begin Stage II and III, but utilize the ketones from you own adipose tissue to help control your appetite.

One final note of caution before beginning the *KetoFast* program. The first few pounds that are lost when any dietary reduction is begun is invariably water, which makes up the largest part of our body weight. The average 160 pound person has almost 100 pounds of body water (50-70% body weight in men, 40-60% in women), mostly intracellular, but nevertheless subject to change when there is a reduction in salt intake. Part of our water stores are contained in a labile compartment that is closely controlled by the intake of salt. When you begin to diet, and reduce the amount of food you are eating, there is a concomitant reduction in the amount of ingested salt. This allows the kidneys to excrete some of the excess water quickly, and the result will show up as a bonafide weight loss which may be encouraging, but is not a sign of long-term success. It is estimated that after one week of fasting, water makes up 40-65% of the total weight loss, with protein making up 5-10%, and fat 30-50%. After one month, however, fat loss accounts for more than 70% of the total weight loss.[47] Athletes who have to reach a designated weight at a particular time, such as wrestlers who are competing at a specific weight limit, have learned that you can easily lose up to ten pounds of this body weight, averaging 2-5% of your total weight through the sweat and diuresis process. Since the water is quickly replaced by altering fluid intake again, little long-term harm is done unless the process is too excessive. This also explains why body wraps will temporarily change the size of your waist or thighs by pressing water out of the intracellular space briefly giving the appearance of weight loss. Given enough time, however, the body will eventually return to the pre-wrap state since nothing has been done to change the actual physiology of the adipose cells. If you want to lose fat, you have to be persistent, which is why *KetoFast* does not return you to normal levels of calorie intake for at least one month.

V. THE *KETOFAST* DIET PROGRAM

The *KetoFast* diet plan is wonderfully simple. There are three Stages which you must complete in order to assure that you can achieve a long-term successful outcome in the management of your weight. In Stage I, you test your metabolism during a total water-fast by measuring the rate at which you burn fat when eliminating all calories from your diet. In essence, this starts your body's ability to burn fat by forcing your enzymes to begin utilizing fatty acids as a fuel source, rather than remaining in a hibernation phase, which is a result of your genetic deficiency of some as yet undefined hormone or enzymatic pathway. In Stage II, you put this process into a stable, continuous mode by maintaining a very-low-calorie diet, which will continue to show ketones periodically in the urine, indicating that you are maintaining fat catabolism as part of your energy source. You are also learning in Stage II how to identify the type and volume of food you can eat to maintain a lowered calorie intake, so that you can successfully continue the process of fat catabolism during Stage III. By ascertaining how to cook your own food, and not relying on premixed meals or portions provided by others, you are able to develop an understanding of how to eat without the assistance of outside professionals. As I have explained throughout this book, your problem with gaining weight is life-long until medical science finds a medication which will cure your deficiency, and it is therefore imperative that you play a primary role in knowing how to manage your food intake. Finally, in Stage III you test your body's ability to achieve a more normal calorie intake, and maintain some fat catabolism, realizing that you will not be able to eat as much food as your friends and neighbors. By increasing your intake of vegetables and reducing your use of calorie-dense foods, you can control your weight without the use of bariatric surgery until medical science provides you with a medication cure.

A. Stage I: The Zero-Calorie Fast

At the beginning of the program, you initiate fat mobilization by undergoing a water-fast until ketones appear in your urine. This phase starts the fires of fat catabolism burning by forcing the body to use up all of its carbohydrate reserves, allowing fat to finally be consumed in the energy-provision process. It requires a total abstinence from all nutrition, except water and vitamins, because of your metabolic deficiency, which has prevented this process from occurring in the past during periods of lowered calorie intake. The duration of Stage I is variable, but typically will last from 2-5 days. You may elect to remain on a water-fast for as long as 1-2 weeks, depending upon your prior experience with the fasting program, but you should check with your physician about any hidden medical problems before extending Stage I beyond 1 week.

25

While you might think that such a regimen is extremely difficult to follow, it is remarkably well-tolerated, since anorexia and euphoria quickly develop once ketosis begins. The association of appetite suppression and starvation is believed to be a compensatory mechanism which has evolved to aid us in times of deprivation, when food is scarce. Most patients will feel some hunger during the first day of the fast, but by the second day it is generally diminished, and by the third day it is usually gone. Alternate-health enthusiasts claim that the feeling of vitality which accompanies a water-fast is due to excess energy being diverted from the necessity of digestion to other bodily functions, especially to the elimination of toxic wastes,[48] but I do not believe that such reasoning is based on physiologic fact. I think that the vigor is more likely due to a diminution in the level of blood sugar elevation which accompanies the eating of food, especially in patients whose calorie intake is high. Even if you are not diabetic, your blood sugar will elevate for at least 2-3 hours after a meal, and this can act as a soporific in many patients. When you are on a water-fast, your blood sugar is derived from the catabolism of glycogen, and sugar levels do not reach the numbers which occur with digestion. When Upton Sinclair underwent his frequent fasts, he noted how he quickly had "that marvellous, abounding energy, so that whenever I had a spare minute or two I would begin to stand on my head, or to 'chin' myself."[49] This type of exhilaration is one reason fasting has become a cultic phenomenon across the globe, not only to lose weight, but to demonstrate the strength of one's inner will-power. Weight loss remains the primary reason to undergo a periodic water-fast, as in the words of Herbert Shelton (1895-1985), a naturopathic physician who was said to have conducted over 30,000 fasts, "there can be no question that fasting produces the quickest, safest and most effective avenue available for weight reduction."[50] This benefit, according to Dr. Allan Cott, who has used fasting to treat thousands of psychiatric patients in New York, is because "the body tolerates a fast better than it does a feast."[51]

Experience with the use of a zero-calorie fast as an effective means of achieving weight loss dates back to the early nineteenth century, when starvation for prolonged periods of time became a public spectacle. A number of individuals, known as "hungerknustlers," even made their living displaying changes in their bodies during prolonged fasts, both for the sake of public display and medical experimentation. In 1908, Dr. Hereward Carrington (1880-1958), PhD, wrote a book extolling the benefits of fasting and outlining the results of his "hunger-cure" or "fasting-cure" of 21 patients. He outlined much of the history of the practice before his time, pointing out that Dr. Martin Luther Holbrook (1831-1902), a well-known medical author and editor, had concluded in 1888 that "fasting is no cunning trick of priestcraft, but the most powerful and safest of all medicines."[52] This reassurance of the benefit of fasting was directed at the belief that no one could fast for an extended period of time and live to tell of it. The 40-day fast of Jesus in the Bible was seen as a miracle, not capable of being safely duplicated by mortal man. It was not until physicians such as Dr. Henry S. Tanner (1831-1919), who described himself as the "father of fasting," underwent similar prolonged fasts for 40 days under close observation that the technique was proven to be not only safe, but therapeutic to the well-being of the patient as well.[53]

With awareness of the effectiveness and safety of the technique of water-fasting came a slew of physicians and scientists who studied the benefits, and presented their findings to the general public in the form of lectures and books. Dr. Edward Hooker Dewey (1839-1904), a practicing physician in Meadville, Pennsylvania, was one of the early proponents of the methodology, extolling the use of fasting to many of his disbelieving colleagues. He so upset his fellow practitioners that he became an outcast, and was asked to submit his resignation from the local medical society. Redirecting his focus of medical care, he became a revered teacher of alternative-health practitioners, and his disciples, as well as many of his famous followers, pointed to his works as educational aids to spread the gospel of the therapeutic water-fast.

Along with the use of frequent water-fasts came recommendations to follow a meat-free vegetarian diet, once food intake was resumed, usually with the use of raw, rather than cooked, vegetables. Professor Arnold Ehret (1866-1922), the father of naturopathy who opened a hugely popular sanitarium in Ascona, Switzerland which he later moved to California, labeled fasting as "Nature's Supreme Remedy," and developed a method of eating which was even more extreme than that recommended by vegetarians. He termed his discovery the "mucusless diet healing system," eliminating all foods except raw and cooked fruits, starchless vegetables, and green-leaf vegetables.[54] Ehret believed that all other foods produced mucous in the body, which was the cause of all of human disease, clogging up the entire excretory system of the body. He came to this conclusion by noting that when potatoes, grain-meal, rice or fat meats were boiled, they give forth a jelly-like slime, which was used as a paste by bookbinders and carpenters. Since digestion is similar to the combustion of boiling, he postulated that this same paste clogged the digestive system and blood.[55] He therefore used fasting to begin the cleansing process, and then initiated his diet to loosen and eliminate the accumulated mucous waste, fasting for periods of 21, 24, 32, and 49 days, all in a period of 14 months, while under close observation to prove his refraining from eating food. His ardent followers became known as "Ehrists," giving rise to the cult of Naturopathy.

One problem with all of these early recommendations to refrain from food for long periods of time was the lack of scientific support for beneficial physiologic effects and safety in carefully controlled experiments. Finally, in

1915, Francis Gano Benedict (1870-1957), a chemist who worked at Wesleyan University in Connecticut, published a book which detailed his research on the metabolic effects of prolonged fasting on an individual who lived in his Nutrition Laboratory for 31 days, eating no food and drinking only distilled water.[56] In that publication, Benedict reviewed the literature on the subject dating back to 1888, summarizing what limited information existed on the physiologic effects of starvation, primarily from studies in Europe.[57] Benedict recorded his findings with meticulous detail, but did not make a judgement on the appropriateness of the use of fasting for weight-loss or medical purposes. He must not have been overly impressed with the efficacy of this method, however, for he changed his focus of inquiry, and in 1919 published with his colleagues at the Carnegie Nutrition Laboratory in Boston a 700-page volume which gave a detailed account of their experiments on the changes in the metabolism of young men during periods of a restricted calorie diet, rather than a water-fast.[58]

Dr. Anton J. Carlson (1875-1976), Professor of Physiology at the University of Chicago, also published data on the benefits of fasting in animals during this early era, having become a devoted faster himself in 1913.[59] With support of efficacy beginning to appear in the medical literature, more advocates began to expound on the benefits of water-fasting as a means of promoting weight loss, as well as ameliorating a multitude of medical diseases. Herbert Shelton, D.C., N.D. (1895-1985) was the most prolific of these enthusiasts, treating over 40,000 patients at his Health School in San Antonio, Texas. His popularity attracted the attention of the medical profession, as well as the state licensing board, resulting in his being arrested, and jailed repeatedly, for practicing medicine without a license.[60] Other medical physicians followed his lead, however, and began to utilize water-fasting as a therapeutic treatment, including Dr. Yuri Nikolayev, director of the fasting unit at the Moscow Psychiatric Institute, who treated over 7,000 patients, achieving a success rate in improving schizophrenia and other neurosis of 70%, a result duplicated by Japanese researchers.[61]

Eventually, the use of fasting as a medical treatment for disease waned, but its benefit as a therapy for obesity was advanced in 1959 by the publication of papers by two researches on opposite sides of the ocean. Dr. Walter Lyon Bloom, from the Ferst Research Center of Piedmont Hospital in Atlanta, published the first modern study of fasting, outlining his treatment of 9 patients, who lost an average of 18 pounds in one week, with some patients losing as much as 2.7 pounds per day.[62] At the same time, Dr. Marian Apfelbaum, from the Hospital X Bichat in Paris, published his results which revealed that patients on a water-fast lost an average of 22 pounds in two weeks, and 50 pounds after fasting for 51 days.[63] These were spectacular results, carried out by respected medical researchers, and the benefits were recognized around the world. Dr. Apfelbaum and Dr. David Benchetrit went on to formulate their diet into a weight-loss program known as leDiet in 1975, and in 2006 their recommendations were the #1 online, self-help diet website, according to a leading U. S. Consumer Advocacy group.[64] One reason for the acceptance of both fasting techniques was the fact that patients were able to easily follow the program, since anorexia uniformly developed within 24 hours, as well as a state of euphoria, which made it easier to stick to the regimen. This prompted Dr. Bloom to declare that "although short periods of total fasting may seem barbaric, this method of reduction is marvelously well tolerated."[65]

As other physicians began to publish their own results of successful weight loss with a prolonged water-fast, the length of time patients were allowed to stay on zero-calories was pushed beyond 1-2 months. One case report from Scotland in 1973 detailed the results of a 382-day fast in a man whose weight dropped from 456 to 180 pounds, an average weight loss of 0.72 pounds per day over the long haul, while other fasts of 350, 256, 249, 236, and 210 days were shown to be tolerated well.[66] Despite the fact that there were consistently high levels of ketones in the urines of these patients, the only significant symptom was occasional lightheadedness. The optimism over the ability to utilize such a prolonged fast to treat morbid obesity was attenuated, however, by the fact that there were occasional fatalities, either during the fast itself, or during the period of refeeding, when the fast lasted more than 1 month.[67] I will discuss how attempts to eliminate the danger of death resulted in an even greater health risk in the next section, but complications were otherwise generally rare, and fasts of less than 1 month duration were shown to be well tolerated.

Despite the fact that many studies have shown that prolonged periods of fasting are quite safe, I do not recommend that patients undergo such treatment without constant supervision by an experienced physician. The *KetoFast* diet does not utilize zero-calorie intake for more than 1-2 weeks to initiate the burning of your fat cells for energy production, and so it is not necessary for you to do any more than get an initial evaluation by your physician, followed by periodic checks if you are on medication for Hypertension or Hypercholesterolemia. If you are on oral medication for Diabetes Mellitus, you should check with your doctor to see if the medication can be withheld during the period of the initial fast, since you could be subject to hypoglycemia if you continued your same dosage. If you are on insulin, you should not undergo a fast without close supervision by an endocrinologist.

Remember that if you actually begin to spill ketones within 24-36 hours of beginning the total caloric fast, you do not need to continue this dietary program, since you are already able to burn fat in the normal fashion, and are not suffering from an hereditary hormone or enzymatic pathway deficiency. Whether you like it or not, you are simply eating too many calories, and you need to learn the proper way to reduce your calorie intake, and increase your expenditure by exercising more often. Feel free to undergo a water-fast for 1-2 days to initiate your weight loss, but your primary problem is that you have made food too much of a social event in your life, and have wallowed in taste sensations for too long, and must now train yourself to eat less. To accomplish this task, you must not prepare or order foods that taste good at the start of your retraining program. It simply is not possible to sit down before a plate of good-looking, good-tasting food, and then eat just a little bit. You must remove the temptation first by removing pleasure from the equation. If you like it rare, make it burnt. If you like it well-done, order it rare. Do not add salt, pepper, garlic, paprika, basil, mustard, etc. No sauces. No taste additives. Take the skin off your chicken and eat it dry. Take the spreads off your bread, and put only lemon or vinegar on your salads. In essence, **if it tastes good, spit it out**. You have already bought this book, so give it to an overweight friend and let that person find out if their own problem is truly organic. Better yet, take advantage of the 100-calorie recipes, and use them rather than fast-foods as snacks. You have still learned something vital about your own metabolism for the purchase price of the book, an investment that will pay you health dividends for the rest of your life.

If your ketones do not appear for over 36 hours, however, proceed to Stage II. Understand one thing: the longer it takes to spill ketones, the more severe is your deficiency. You will have to spend more time stoking the fires of fat-catabolism if you are going to achieve long-lasting weight control, so be prepared to spend the time necessary for altering your metabolic system. Although most patients will begin to spill ketones by the third day and may elect to immediately enter Stage II, you can remain on a water-fast safely for up to 7-10 days, but the longer you remain on a fast, the more important it is to break the fast with liquid juices for the first day or two, since peristalsis of the stomach may be delayed in responding to the digestion of food. Advocates who fast for weeks at a time have elaborate suggestions for how to break a prolonged water-fast, but for the purposes of the *KetoFast* diet, you should not have a problem as long as you do not fast for longer than 7-10 days. The key to success is in learning how your own body works, and then designing a dietary plan to control your genetic deficiency until some type of medical aide is available in the years to come. Don't get angry. Don't get frustrated. And most of all, don't say you can't do it, because you can lose weight if you truly make the effort to train your body to accept the caloric limitations which control the production of fat.

B. Stage II: The Very-Low-Calorie Diet (VLCD)

As mentioned above, although a prolonged water-fast was found to be very effective in causing profound weight loss, occasional deaths were reported in the medical literature when the fast lasted longer than 1 month. Because the ingestion of only water is known to be associated with significant protein loss and muscle wasting, as manifested by a negative nitrogen balance with excessive excretion of nitrogen in the urine, it was surmised early on that these fatalities could have been due to heart muscle damage, resulting in a disruption of cardiac muscle contractility, and secondary fatal cardiac arrhythmias. A number of investigators therefore began to study the substitution of a very-low calorie diet (VLCD), below 600 calories a day, for zero-calorie fasting as a means to attenuate the loss of protein. Frank Evans, James Strang, and H. B. McClugage, from Western Pennsylvania Hospital in Pittsburgh, published a series of papers between 1929-1931 showing that a VLCD of 360 calories could be maintained at home for up to 6 months, with patients losing an average of 2.5 pounds per week over the long-haul, and over 4 pounds per week at the beginning of the diet.[68] These results may not have been as imposing as the 1-2 pounds per day which occurred with a zero-calorie diet, but it was still a very impressive outcome. Not only was the VLCD successful in causing significant weight loss, but the patients felt quite well, often to the point of euphoria, and complained of minimal hunger, similar to the situation with a water-fast.[69] Although the diet was radical at the time, causing them to label their initial paper "A Departure from the Usual Methods in Treating Obesity," their suggestions would not be considered extreme today, as a typical daily menu consisted of 1 egg and 1-ounce of bread for breakfast, 1 egg and 4-ounces of vegetable for lunch, and 1 cup bouillon, 3-ounces lean meat, and 4-ounces of vegetable for dinner.[70]

It is not known how many people may have been treated with this regimen, since the authors never followed up their research in the medical press, but the technique never became commercialized, and the concept was set aside until the British endocrinologist Dr. T. W. Simeons resurrected the idea in 1954, with his "Simeons diet," a program consisting of an intake of 575 calories/day for 6 weeks, supplemented by daily injections of human chorionic gonadotrophin (HCG). Simeons claimed that the injections were necessary for the dietary success, and charged handsomely for his services in his clinic in Rome, but subsequent studies clearly showed that HCG provided no more weight loss than saline injections, so most critics believe that it was the motivation of daily attendance that likely kept his patients on schedule, assuring a successful weight loss.[71] This same motivation has likely helped companies like Weight Watchers and Jenny Craig assure their clients that weight loss will occur if they maintain a good attendance record.

The profit motives of Simeons was not lost on other entrepreneurs, and commercial products soon became available in the 1960s to reproduce the low-calorie menu with a powder that could be easily mixed with water and ingested daily, assuring that adequate calorie-restriction was maintained. In order to try and reduce the 4-5 gms of nitrogen lost in the urine each day with the standard VLCD, these supplements added extra amounts of protein to help prevent excessive muscle catabolism. The first commercial diet of this type was Metrocal, a product of Mead Johnson which became available in supermarkets in 1962, and contained 900 calories per day, more than that supplied by the VLCDs. It was intended to be the sole source of nutrition, and was nutritionally complete. Because a patient was not allowed to eat any other type of food, it assured adherence, and was successful in causing significant weight loss. The process was monotonous and unpalatable, however, leading to a very high drop-out rate, and the product was eventually withdrawn from the market place.

Robert Bolinger and his colleagues at the University of Kansas Medical Center in 1966,[72] and the program headed by Marian Apfelbaum, at Hospital X Bichat in Paris, France in 1967,[73] further advanced the concept of protein-sparing, low-calorie formulas by utilizing high-quality protein supplements, as well as vitamins, minerals, and trace elements. Bolinger used egg whites as his protein source, while Apfelbaum used milk proteins, from which lipids and lactose had been carefully removed. Both achieved weight losses that averaged 50-80% of the starvation fast, and their technique became known as a "protein-supplemented fast."[74] The advantage of losing fat, rather than lean muscle tissue, spurred a plethora of commercially available liquid protein supplements, which were of much lower grade than that used by these two groups. In order to lower costs, and make a product to satisfy large numbers of people, hydrolyzed gelatin or collagen was used as the protein source, even though it was deficient in several essential amino acids, as well as vital vitamins and minerals.[75] The popularity of these "liquid protein" diets rapidly increased following the publication of *The Last Chance Diet* by Linn and Stuart in 1976, and more than 100,000 people used these diets exclusively for at least one month in 1977.[76] Although the weight loss was spectacular, it was ultimately shown that at least 17 deaths (16 women and 1 man) occurred in 1977 and 1978 among patients using the supplements as their sole calorie source,[77] with all of the deaths taking place after at least two months of use, and loss of 30-35% of body weight.[78]

Needless to say, there was an immediate reaction from the government and physicians alike to pull these ill-conceived products off the market, and medical research soon identified the lack of adequate supplementation of vitamins, minerals and carbohydrates, along with a poor protein base, as the root cause. Modifications were quickly made to the formulas, and two acceptable formats soon became available, including the Optifast diet (pioneered by Genuth and Vertes and distributed by Novartis Pharmaceutical), introduced in 1974, and the Cambridge diet (a flavored powder mixed with water and consumed three times daily, totaling 330 calories), introduced in 1980.[79] These two products became very successful in both the United States and Europe, and the Optifast diet, in particular, received widespread publicity when Oprah Winfrey divulged to 18 million viewers in 1988 that she lost 67 pounds in 4 months using the Optifast formula.[80]

Although these formulations were gaining ready acceptance by the general public as a weight-loss aid throughout the world, they were still considered radical by some medical practitioners, and to help evaluate their results and safety record, a continuum of meetings of experts in the field were held, including the Life Sciences Research Office of the Federation of American Societies of Experimental Biology and Medicine in 1970, the Third International Congress on Obesity in 1980, and a Symposium on Very Low Calorie Diets meeting in 1983. Part of the reason for calling these meetings was the rapid growth of the usage of these diets, particularly the Cambridge Diet, which was said to have been used by 5 million persons between 1980-1982.[81] An edited version of the papers presented at the Symposium on Very Low Calorie Diets was published by George L. Blackburn and George A. Bray in 1985, entitled *Management of Obesity by Severe Caloric Restriction*. The general consensus of the participants was that VLCDs (400-800 calories per day) which utilized poor quality protein were dangerous, but those which used high quality protein, along with vitamin and mineral supplementation, had a good safety record and were an acceptable way to lose weight.[82] These opinions supporting the use of VLCDs to lose weight were confirmed by Alan H. Howard, PhD, Director of the Lipid Laboratory at Cambridge University's Addenbrooke's Hospital, who corroborated the conclusion that semisynthetic diets in the region of 250 calories per day could be used safely over periods of up to one year.[83] Once professional backing for the use of VLCDs was confirmed, their sales increased, and by 2001, over 25 million people had followed such diets and there was "no evidence of pathological changes as a result."[84] In addition to a good safety record, the effectiveness of the VLCDs matched that of the earlier studies, with weight loss averaging 3.3 pounds (1.5 kg) per week in women, and 4.4 pounds (2.2 kg) per week in men.[85]

So why am I not simply telling you to close this book at this stage and go buy a year's worth of pre-fab food to take inches from your waist? The answer lies in the fact that these diets are artificially prepared powders that never teach you what kind of food you have to eat in order to maintain your lower weight for the rest of your life. There is no question that if you stick to one of these rigidly controlled artificial diets, you will lose weight. VLCDs are effective, and safe. If you are overweight because of excessive eating, this may be all you need to maintain a lower weight. Start your weight loss rapidly with one of these programs, and then learn to control your calorie intake to reasonable levels.

But because of your genetic disorder, your problem is more intense, and may not be controllable with calorie-intake levels that work for your neighbors and friends. You will immediately begin to regain weight as soon as you switch to eating normal foods, unless you have learned how to evaluate how many calories you can eat to maintain a relatively normal weight. The VLCD diets are fine for the short-term, but you cannot rely on restricting your intake in this manner forever. That is why the *KetoFast* diet is a much better method of losing weight, since you eat the same number of calories as the VLCDs, but you learn how to eat smaller portions of food, both at home and when you are on the road. By periodically checking your urine for ketones, and utilizing the recipes in this book, you can estimate how many calories are included in menu items at a restaurant, and learn how to practice portion-control. This is a necessary part of any long-term weight management program, but it is vitally important to you, and can only be successful by a hands-on approach.

Stage II of *KetoFast* teaches you how to search for a calorie intake level that will allow you to continue to lose weight, while at the same time adjusting the flame of your metabolic system. Despite the supportive evidence of safety in the medical literature, it is still possible that allowing ketone levels to remain at a high level for prolonged periods of time could lead to deleterious alterations in your normal physiologic function. While weight loss would be more rapid, so would potential health complications. At the same time, if you turn off your catabolism of fat at too early of a stage, your body will enter a hibernation mode, and weight loss will cease. The object of *KetoFast* is to regulate the amount of fat you burn by providing some outside calorie source, while fine-tuning the production of energy from your adipose tissue. You accomplish this by adding 100-calorie increments of food in Stage II, while checking the ketones in your urine to assure that some fat catabolism is taking place. The duration of this Stage is variable, but will usually last from 6-8 weeks. You should not end this Stage until you have lost 10-15% of your normal body weight, and feel comfortable that you have enough control over your appetite to immediately reign in any excess desire to eat larger volumes of food.

Because the calories are added in 100-calorie increments, all of the recipes in this book are in the 100-calorie range, allowing you to vary your food intake by choosing foods you would prefer to eat. The choice of food is yours, as I do not believe the type of calorie is important -- be it carbohydrate, protein, or fat -- but you must not increase your total calorie intake in Stage II above 600 calories per day. As you add the 100-calorie portions, you should spread them throughout the day by first eating a portion for dinner, and then adding one at lunch 2 days later, and finally one more, 2 days later, for breakfast. From this point, continue to add 100-calories every 2-3 days, either by taking portions between meals and at bedtime, or by increasing the amount you eat three times a day, never increasing any one meal above 200 calories. You do not increase your total caloric intake unless you have shown some ketone production during the day. If no ketones appear in the urine for more than two days, lower your calorie intake by 100 calories for another two days. Many patients find that it is better to eat six 100-calorie portions a day instead of three 200-calorie meals, as this will help prevent insulin surges which can accentuate your hunger, and decrease your burning of fat. In addition, as you get used to eating smaller portions in this Stage, it will assist you in keeping your total calorie intake low when you enter Stage III.

Some health enthusiasts have recommended that you not eat breakfast, and only begin your intake of food later in the day, when your hunger increases. This was a particularly prominent argument of Hereward Carrington in 1908, who cautioned his readers to "omit the breakfast," since there is no natural hunger in the morning after a restful night's sleep, and there has been no expenditure of energy to require replacement by the ingestion of food.[86] I do not have a major problem with this suggestion once you are eating more than 600 calories per day, but I believe that you will be better able to maintain a stable insulin output during Stage II by eating at least 3 times per day. This will also allow you to evaluate your ketone excretion closely, and delay intake of food if ketones disappear from more than 3 consecutive urine specimens.

It is not necessary to purposely increase your ingestion of protein in order to reduce muscle catabolism, as it has been clearly shown that eating carbohydrates will reduce the catabolism of protein more effectively than increasing the ingestion of protein.[87] As will be discussed shortly, if you think that low glycemic foods are better for you, feel free to utilize them in your own diet plan. If you want to eat only vegetables and no animal protein, be my guest. As long as you show intermittent ketones in your urine, your system is burning fat, and your ability to lose weight is assured. Realize, however, that some degree of protein ingestion is necessary, so try and supplement your meals with vegetables and grains that have high amounts of protein, such as oatmeal, dried peas, nuts, and beans, especially soy products.

I want to stress that this may be your most difficult phase to handle, since hunger can become a more prominent feature in Stage II than in Stage I. As discussed above, it is common for people on a fast to not become very hungry. Once you introduce 100-calorie portions, however, the smell, taste, and look of food will accentuate your desire to eat larger portions. You can make an effort to control your desires if you remember that the testing of your urine is proof of how successful you can be, and how wrong others have been to blame your weight on eating larger portions of food. With time, your appetite will be controllable, but at the start you must have faith, and believe in yourself, sticking to the smaller portions until your loss of weight allows you to progress into Stage III.

C. Stage III: Moderate Calorie Control

Once you have reached a level of stable weight loss, which generally means you have lost 10-15% of your initial body weight, you can then begin to gradually increase your calorie intake above 600 calories per day, attempting to reach a level of 1000-1200 calories per day for at least another 2 months. Because of your physiologic condition, the likelihood that future weight gain will recur is great, and you must therefore assure that you maintain a mechanism by which fat cells can be quickly catabolized. This is accomplished by keeping your "pilot light" of fat catabolism lit through a process of water-fasting for 24 hours every 1-2 weeks, in order to minimize your body's storage of glycogen. You must check your urine for ketones during this period of time, and make sure that you are able to spill at least a trace amount of ketone. Since the average BMR is in this same calorie range of 1000-1200 calories per day, you should be able to catabolize some fat, and not return to your previously deficient state utilizing this method, but it is not possible to easily measure your BMR, and it is possible that you will need to maintain a lower than normal calorie intake. While Stage III may actually last your entire life span, or at least until medical science discovers the causation of your obesity, you will at least be able to remain at a reasonable level of weight by periodically checking for ketone excretion in your urine. To eventually increase your total daily calorie intake to more normal levels, you will have to raise your daily expenditure of calories by exercise, as will be discussed shortly.

Do not listen to those "experts" who claim that it is outside of your nature to eat only 1200 calories per day for long periods of time. In the sixteenth century, Louis Cornaro (1464-1566), a Venetian nobleman, wrote a book entitled *Discourses on the Sober Life*, which outlined his method for living to the ripe old age of 102. At age 40, after living a reckless and dissipated life, Cornaro limited himself to twelve ounces of solid food daily, along with fourteen ounces of light wine, a regimen which he continued for the rest of his life.[88] His story has been cited by many alternative-health advocates as evidence of the value of reducing the amount of food we eat, in order to prevent an overload of our digestive system. While no single case report defines the needs of most people, rest assured that you can learn to live quite well, and quite satisfied, with a lower volume of food intake, especially if you utilize low calorie-dense foods, such as raw vegetables. The main reason people today still think that higher calorie intakes are necessary for good health stems from the studies of physicians in the late 19th and early 20th centuries, which claimed that most working men needed more than 3000 calories per day to maintain a strong constitution. The Munich physiologist, Carl Voit (1831-1908), studied laborers who consumed approximately 3100 calories daily, and concluded that protein intake for people should be 118 grams per day, a value that became known as the "Voit standard."[89] Other so-called experts followed with similar recommendations, and the general belief became ingrained that in order to increase muscle mass and stamina, one had to eat large amounts of meat. This assessment was shattered by Dr. Russell Henry Chittenden (1856-1943), professor of physiological chemistry and Directory of the Sheffield Scientific School at Yale University from 1822-1922, who subjected the study of protein intake to scientific scrutiny and conclusively showed that the recommendations were greatly exaggerated. His studies proved that a man of average weight only required 0.12 gm of nitrogen per kilogram of body-weight, about 60 grams of protein a day, one-half the amount in the Voit standard.[90] He clearly showed that one did not have to eat a high proportion of protein to increase vitality, and that military men who ate a high carbohydrate meal, rather than their more typical high meat-protein meal, increased, rather than decreased, their physical strength, while maintaining their weight at a more desirable level.[91] Not only was the ingestion of high amounts of protein unnecessary, it was also dangerous and could lead to "gastro-intestinal disturbance, indigestion, intestinal toxemia, liver roubles, bilious attacks, gout, rheumatism, to say nothing of many other ailments."[92] This supported the view of Hereward Carrington, who warned years before that "the majority of people are eating two or three times as much as they need, and the consequence is that they cannot utilize it all, and it accumulates in the body as half-burned material," resulting not only in accumulation of adipose tissue, but in protein waste.[93]

Chittenden's research spawned a new theory of healthy nutrition, which claimed that illnesses were due to "poisonous congestion," brought about by eating large amounts of food which went beyond the body's need for maintenance."[94] Such damage would occur by both an improper selection of animal-based foods ("proteid" foods), and an excess supply, the overeating of which "produces auto-intoxication, self-poisoning, malassimilation, premature old age or disease - call it what you will."[95] As concluded by Chittenden, protein catabolism yields "a row of crystalline nitrogenous products," which exercises "more or less of a deleterious influence upon the system."[96] Although Chittenden's work was seminal in improving our understanding of the dangers of eating too much meat, his promotion of carbohydrates and fat likely led to our populations gradual accumulation of weight, since eating carbohydrates at calorie-levels greater than that used in his subjects will promote weight-gain. The Western diet became over-saturated with calories in all three food groups, and the resultant rise in obesity is what has necessitated the publication of this book.

The advantage of lower calorie intakes is not only evident in human beings, but throughout the animal kingdom, as well. Dr. Roy L. Walford (1924-2004) and his colleagues at the University of California in Los Angeles (UCLA) showed that mice who were fed 50% of their normal calorie intake, but maintained nutritional requirements, more than doubled their expected life span.[97] This benefit existed "across nearly the whole animal kingdom," with changes in cholesterol, fasting glucose, insulin levels, and other parameters of health mimicking that seen in humans.[98] Walford referred to his suggestions as the calorie restriction with optimal nutrition (CRON) diet, a term which was popularized into the "120 Year Diet" and the "Anti-Aging Plan" in the press.[99]

Many individuals feel extremely energized and proud of their accomplishments by ingesting no food for 24 hours, but if you do not want to revert to a water-fast in Stage III, you can elect to go on a 2-3 day fruit and vegetable juice-fast, which allows the intake of fresh juice preparations, but not solid food. Sometimes referred to as "liquitarianism," this type of diet is widely used by alternate health-care advocates across the globe for as long as 30 days, and is claimed to speed the elimination of toxins, such as artificial colors, flavors, preservatives, pesticides, insecticides, and rancid oils from the body by redirecting the energy that is used to digest solid foods into a cleansing of the body organs. Proof of this toxin-cleansing, often labeled as a "healing crisis," "cleansing reaction," or "Herxheimer reaction," is said to be the explanation for symptoms such as nausea, exhaustion, diarrhea, muscle aches, nervousness, shortness of breath, coating of the tongue, bad breath, body odor, excess mucus from your sinuses, and skin eruptions, which frequently accompany a prolonged juice-fast.[100] Arnold Ehret labeled the coating of the tongue as the "magic mirror," which enabled fasters to tell how many toxins were being excreted from their body.[101]

Proponents of juice-fasts claim that the diet boosts your immune system, improves liver function, and even provides large amounts of oxidative enzymes, which not only helps to prevent cancer, but can treat patients with medical diseases as well.[102] I am not convinced of the reliability of these claims, but it is clear that we are all exposed to an enormous array of toxins from many diverse sources. Around the world, there are now over 100,000 synthetic chemicals on the market, which enter our bodies from the food we eat, the air we breathe, and the water we drink.[103] Data from the U.S. in 1989

38

indicated that more than 6 billion tons of waste were produced annually, averaging nearly 50,000 pounds per resident person,[104] and Canadian researchers have pointed to the fact that industries in Canada admitted releasing 20,343 tons of known carcinogens into the air, soil, and water in 2001, resulting in the fact that 41% of Canadian males and nearly 38% of females will develop some form of cancer.[105] In the United States these figures are even higher, with males having a more than 47% chance of developing cancer in 1998, and females a 38% chance, percentages which continue to rise each year. Absorption of these chemical toxins is so ubiquitous that it has been estimated that anyone willing to put up $2,000 to have their body tested would discover at least 250 dangerous chemical contaminants.[106]

Some of the most prevalent toxins which contaminate our system are lead, from industrial processes, pesticide sprays, paint and cooking utensils; mercury, from dental fillings and contaminated fish (especially Mackerel, Shark, Swordfish, and Tilefish); aluminum, from antacids, cookware, and soda cans; industrial chemicals, such as PCBs (production banned in 1976, but not until 1,700,000 tons had already been loosed into the environment); phenol, from cleaning products; formaldehyde, from paints, new carpets and furniture; polycyclic aromatic hydrocarbons (PAHs), from auto exhaust, factory smoke stacks, petroleum tar products and tobacco smoke; pesticides, including DDT (restricted by the Environmental Protection Agency in 1972), chlordane, lindane, aldrin, dieldrin, endrin, toxaphene, heptachlor, and dioxin (the most potent carcinogen ever tested in animal species, and a contaminant of Agent Orange), all put at the top of the danger list by Rachel Carson in *Silent Spring* in 1962; microbial toxins, from a variety of food products; chlorine, from our drinking water; nitrites, used as a meat preservative and color and flavor enhancer, especially in hot dogs, bacon and canned meats, capable of being converted into carcinogenic nitrosamines; nonylphenols, from plastic containers, wraps and personal care products; and bisphenol-A, from hard plastic water bottles (recently banned by Canada in baby bottles), DVDs, and CDs, just to name a few. Secondary cigarette smoke is a significant source of toxin exposure, filling the air with cadmium, cyanide, lead, arsenic, tars, radioactive material, dioxin, carbon monoxide, hydrogen cyanide, nitrogen oxides, nicotine, sulfur oxides, and about 4,000 other chemicals.[107] Vegetarians may claim that there are many health benefits from avoiding meat-products, but they are also exposed to a high pesticide load, even if they routinely wash the vegetables before consumption. According to the Environmental Working Group, the products which have the highest concentration of chemicals are peaches, apples, sweet bell peppers, celery, nectarines, strawberries, cherries, lettuce, imported grapes, and pears, in decreasing order of danger.[108] With such an incredible load of contamination in our environment, it is no wonder that the human species is experiencing a rising incidence of cancer, but the danger also effects our future progeny, since studies have shown that the effective sperm count of men across the world has been lowered by 50%, a result blamed on the rising levels of toxic chemicals in our system.[109]

Many proponents of fasting have claimed that the only way to rid your system of these dangerous substances is to modify your diet to ingest only water or juice, and thereby funnel your energy into toxic cleansing, rather than digestion. That fasts can reduce the damage from chemical exposure has been shown by their attenuation of symptoms in sixteen patients who were poisoned by ingesting rice oil contaminated with polychlorobiphenyls (PCBs) in Taiwan.[110] While I do not believe that this detoxification effect is a significant health benefit in all patients, I do accept that this type of program, used periodically, will allow you to assure that you are able to burn fat quickly, once you begin to increase your calorie intake, and possibly assist in the reduction of certain chemicals that may have accumulated in your body. Overweight patients are at greater risk for damage by toxins of this type, since chemicals usually accumulate in adipose tissue.

That leakage of toxins from fat cells into the circulation can seriously impair the health of humans was what prompted L. Ron Hubbard (1911-1986), the founder of the Church of Scientology, to develop his purification (detoxification) procedure for patients who were suffering from lysergic acid diethylamide (LSD) disorders in 1977.[111] LSD was a popular psychedelic drug in the mid-twentieth century, becoming a favorite of Hippies around the world who were searching for states of intoxication. They were encouraged in this behavior by advocates like Dr. Timothy Leary (1920-1996) and Dr. Richard Alpert, who claimed that LSD could lead to spiritual growth. Because LSD lodged in the fatty tissue when it was first ingested, it could leach out years later and cause reactions which made it appear that the individual had just taken LSD again. In order to cleanse the system of all remnants of the drug, as well as other addictive substances, Hubbard developed his "sweat program," which utilized daily exercise (20-30 minutes of running), a 3-4 ½ hour sauna, and vitamin and nutrient supplementation to sweat out the accumulated toxins for at least a 3-4 week period of time.[112] The purpose of the running was to acclerate the blood circulation in order to pump out the impurities, and then dispel it into the sweat with the sauna. Vitamins and minerals had to be taken in sufficient quantities to replace those washed out by the sweating.[113] Soy, walnut, peanut and safflower oil were ingested in order to exchange the bad toxin-infested fat in the body for good oil.[114] His 5-hour daily routine was extremely strenuous, but it worked, and is used today in clinics around the world to aid in addiction withdrawal from a number of substances. While Hubbard's intense program should not be attempted by overweight patients simply trying to lose weight, the underlying theory of detoxification is similar to those who propose a water- or juice-fast, and it is possible that some benefit may accrue to those who elect to undergo the *KetoFast* diet.

One advantage of incorporating periodic juice-fasting into Stage III is that it can assist you in refraining from falling into bad eating habits, which may have helped get you into your obese condition in the first place. When you restrict your intake to liquids alone, you do not chew your food, which stimulates the secretion of digestive juices and increases your hunger. While chewing gum may help you smoke fewer cigarettes, it is not advantageous if you want to reduce your appetite. By going on a juice-fast, you will be able to lower your calorie intake, especially if you dilute the juice with equal parts of water.

Vegetables commonly used in juice-fasts include alfalfa (rich in chlorophyll), bean sprouts, beets (powerful liver regenerator), bell pepper, broccoli, cabbage, carrots (rich in vitamin A and all the essential minerals and vitamins), celery (excellent source of organic sodium, magnesium and iron, and a strong kidney tonic), chard, cucumber (rich in potassium, iron and magnesium), dandelion greens (rich in magnesium), green peppers, endive, head lettuce, kale (high in carotenes, chlorophyll and calcium), parsley (strong taste, high chlorophyll), potatoes (high in potassium and sulfur), radishes (high in mineral content), red tomatoes (rich in vegetable amino acids), romaine lettuce (rich in magnesium, iron and chlorophyll), string beans (good for diabetics), sweet spinach, sweet potatoes, turnip leaves (high in calcium and vitamin C), watercress (high in sulfur), wheatgrass, and zucchini. Fruits most frequently utilized are apples, blueberries, cantaloupe (considered by many the most nutritious of all fruits), grapes, grapefruits, lemons (rich in bio-flavonoids), oranges, pears, pineapples, strawberries, and watermelons (including the rind). Dr. H. E. Kirschner, a practicing physician and author of *Live Food Juices*, is noted for his use of carrot juice, which he claims helped one woman reclaim her health shortly after she began taking one gallon of carrot juice a day for 18 months, without ingesting any other solid or liquid food. Another one of his patients claimed to have lived only on carrot juice and the solids from goat whey for 4 ½ years.[115] These examples are not necessarily to be accepted at face value, or recommended for general use, but they do point out that radically limited food intake can sustain good health for long periods of time.

If you do decide to follow a juice diet, there are certain precautions you should take to assure that you reduce your exposure to pesticides and bacteria as much as possible. Always remove the skins of oranges, lemons, and grapefruits because of contamination with chemicals used in the growth and transportation process, but it is safe to leave the white pithy part of the peel.

You should also remove all pits, and apple seeds, although seeds from lemons, lime, melons and grapes can be retained. In general, you cannot get adequate amounts of juice from the pulp of apricot, avocado, banana, coconut meat, papaya, peach or strawberry, but some advocates recommend the use of these products anyway, since they are nutritious and tasty. Collard greens, dandelion greens and mustard greens are also very beneficial, but are bitter-tasting and should be used sparingly. Cabbage is an excellent cleansing agent, but bacteria in the gut may break down the fiber into a foul smelling gas, so consider your social obligations before ingesting this product.

To reduce bacterial contamination, fill your sink with cold water and add either 4 tablespoons of salt and ½ cup of white vinegar, or the juice from 3 lemons, or 1 teaspoon of Clorox bleach, or 1 tablespoon of 35%, food-grade hydrogen peroxide. Soak the fruits and vegetables for 10 minutes, and then rinse thoroughly with cold water. It is better to undertake this tedious process and make the juices fresh, then to use bottled juices, most of which have been pasteurized, leading to the loss of many of the enzymes and phytonutrients during the process and long storage on the grocery shelf.

Herbs, such as parsley, cilantro, yucca root, fennel, spearmint, peppermint, basil, ginger, garlic, green onion, chile pepper, turmeric root, and milk thistle may also be utilized, both for their taste and health benefits. A quick drink which is extremely low in calories can be simply prepared by adding 2 tablespoons of raw, unfiltered apple-vinegar to a large glass of water. This adds only 30 calories to your daily calorie total, but other juice products will have to be assessed for their contribution. An 8-ounce glass of juice will contain the following calories: apple, 125 calories; beet, 110 calories; carrot, 108 calories; celery 45 calories; cucumber, 42 calories; grape, 231 calories; grapefruit, 100 calories; lemon, 105 calories; lettuce, 47 calories; orange, 132 calories; pineapple, 103 calories; spinach 58 calories; and tomato, 56 calories.[116] If you dilute the juices with water, your calorie intake will be lowered, so let your taste determine how much dilution can be tolerated.

Finally, I do not believe that the acidity of your food has any importance in following the *KetoFast* diet, but if you believe in the *Acid-Alkaline Diet* promoted by Christopher Vasey, you should avoid utilizing tomatoes, eggplant, nectarines, strawberries, raspberries, lemons, oranges, grapefruit, and pineapples in the recipes listed below, and should dilute your juices with alkaline mineral water.[117] Once you complete the weight loss phase of your program, you can consider reducing your intake of acidic foods as desired.

To prepare your own juice-fast favorites, all you need is a good juice extractor (not a blender). The juices should be consumed as soon as they are prepared, or shortly thereafter, since vegetable juice is one of the most perishable foods, and should not be kept for more than 24 hours in an air-tight container in the refrigerator. The juices should always be ingested at room temperature, and the average serving is 10-12 ounces, although you can take up to 16 ounces if you wish. For fruit juices alone, you may add ice and blend into a smoothie if desired. If you ardently believe in the detoxification process, utilize only organic, pesticide-free produce, but for the purposes of the *KetoFast* diet this extra cost is not necessary.

The use of only one particular food or fruit juice to aid in the loss of weight is known as a "mono diet." The benefits are supposedly due to the fact that the digestive process is simplified by requiring enzymes to be secreted against only one food type, allowing nutritive substances to be quickly absorbed so that energy can be diverted to the elimination of toxins (autolysis), as in a water-fast.[118] One of the most popular of these techniques was the so-called "Hollywood Diet," or "Mayo Clinic Diet," although it was never endorsed by the Mayo Clinic. It utilized only grapefruit juice, which was chosen because it provides little sugar load, and reduces insulin levels in the blood. Grapefruit juice was used as a sole supplement throughout the day, in a fashion similar to the water-fast, and in the 1933 comedy movie "Hard to Handle," James Cagney's character Lefty dreamt up an 18-day Grapefruit Diet as a way to back his investors. Bottled versions of this product are still available today, combining the grapefruit with other supposedly healthy ingredients, but in my opinion, if you want to utilize grapefruit alone for a short period of time, you can save money by simply adding multivitamin tablets as supplementation. Lemon juice acts in a similar manner and can be taken liberally by mixing the juice of ½-1 lemon in a glass of water. These options will provide you with an alternative to a water-fast during the few times you need to check your ability to spill ketones in the urine.

Another mono diet which has achieved acclaim in the past is the "Grape Cure," which was acclaimed by Johanna Brandt in 1928 of curing her stomach cancer. The grape is known to have diuretic and laxative properties, and also a stimulant effect on the liver to neutralize and destroy toxins. In addition, it has numerous vitamins and mineral, and even a small amount of protein, while containing only 100 calories per 1 2/3 cup. Although these attributes are not to be expected to cure cancer, it is possible that they can aid in weight loss. Brandt suggested that between 1-4 pounds of grapes be taken daily, for up to 2 months, and then followed by a diet of raw fruits and vegetables.[119] Other mono diets which have been used toward this same purpose include the Breuss vegetable juice cure (celery, beet, potato, black radish), developed by the Austrian naturopath Rudolf Breuss, the macrobiotic brown rice diet, and the dried apricot diet of the Hunza in northern Pakistan.[120]

43

Most juice-enthusiasts prefer mixtures of fruits and vegetables,
however, and some of the more popular combinations include:

2 apples, 1 cucumber 1 large kale leaf

2 apples, 2 celery stalks, 1/2 ounce ginger juice

2 apples, 2 tomatoes, 1 clove garlic, sprig of parsley

2 apples, 2 celery stalks, 2 carrots

2 apples, 2 carrots, 1 sweet potato, one thin slice Spanish onion,
pinch of dulse powder

½ avocado, 1 tomato, 1 red or green pepper, and 3 leaves of spinach
or cabbage

1 beet, 2 yams, 1 slice Spanish onion, 2 lemons, 1 celery stalk, small
slice of ginger

1 beet, 2 radishes, 1 lemon, 1 slice Spanish onion, 2 sweet potatoes, 1
celery stalk, 2 tablespoons cider vinegar

1 beet, 1 sweet potato, 2 apples, 1 lemon, 1 tomato, 1 garlic clove

1 beet, 1 carrot, 1 celery stalk, ½ potato, 1 radish (Rudolf Breuss's
anticancer mixture)

1 beet, 2 carrots, 2 celery stalks, ½ sweet potato

1 beet, 3 carrots, ½ bunch parsley, 2 celery stalks, 1/4 head cabbage,
1 apple

1 beet, 3 carrots, 1 ounce baby spinach, 2 celery stalks; ½ cantaloupe,
2 pears, 1 inch piece of fresh ginger root

1 cup broccoli, ½ bunch parsley, 2 celery stalks, 1 cucumber, 1/4
head cabbage, 1 bell pepper, 1 lemon

1 cup broccoli, 4 medium tomatoes, 2 celery stalks, ½ cucumber, 1
clove garlic

1 cup broccoli, 2 tomatoes, 2 stalks celery, ½ green pepper, 1 clove
garlic

½ small red cabbage, ½ fennel bulb, 2 apples, 1 tablespoon lemon
juice

5 carrots, 3 celery stalks, 1 small beet

4 carrots, 2 tomatoes, 2 stalks celery, 1 handful spinach

2 celery stalks, ½ cucumber, 1 large kale leaf, ½ cup spinach, 1
radish, small sprig parsley

1 green pepper, 1 red pepper, 3 celery stalks, ½ cucumber, 5 lettuce
leaves.

1 kale leaf, 1 collard leaf, small handful of parsley, 1 celery stalk, 1
carrot, ½ red pepper, 1 tomato, 1 broccoli floret

1 orange, 1 hard pear, 1 yam, 1 grapefruit, 1 apple

4 oranges, 1 pineapple, 1 sweet potato

3 tomatoes, ½ green or red pepper, 1 celery stalk, 1 apple, ½ teaspoon
onion powder, ½ teaspoon garlic powder, 1 teaspoon
Worcestershire sauce, pinch of freshly ground black
powder

3 tomatoes, ½ bunch cilantro, 1 fresh mild jalapeno, 1 sweet red
pepper, 2 celery stalks, ½ sweet onion

½ tomato, 1/4 cucumber, 1 carrot, 1 celery stalk, 1 handful spinach, ½
red pepper, ½ cup cabbage, 1 green onion, 1/8 teaspoon sea
salt
1 wedge watermelon with rind, ½ pound red grapes

Finally, I want to mention a variant of the fruit juice mixture, which has been developed to aid in the cleansing of the gastrointestinal (GI) tract. Stanley Burroughs (1903-1991), an alternative-health practitioner who was convicted of second-degree murder in California for his unauthorized medical treatments, utilized a special lemonade mixture he termed the "Master Cleanser," consisting of the juice of ½ lemon (2 tablespoons), 2 tablespoons of genuine maple syrup (Grade B or C), and 1/10 teaspoon (pinch) of cayenne pepper (to help wash out the mucous loosened by the cleanse), with 10 ounces of medium-hot spring or purified water (cold is acceptable), taken every 1-2 hours throughout the day along with purified water.[121] Since maple syrup contains 52 calories per tablespoon, and one lemon has about 20 calories, a glass of this product would add about 110 calories. Although Burroughs did not recommend any other foods or drinks during the 10-30 days one remained on this diet, leading to the conviction for murder mentioned above, many followers today still utilize his lemonade mixture as a cathartic aid, resulting in his book, *The Master Cleanser*, ranking #170 in sales at Amazon.com in 2007.[122] I do not recommend that you follow Burrough's directive to take this one product throughout the day as your only source of caloric intake, but utilizing the Master Cleanser during Stage II and III as one of your 100-calorie portions to aid in the defecation process, is acceptable. A similar drink, which totals only about 85 calories, can be mixed by adding the juice of 2-3 ounces of fresh ginger root, 1/4 lime, 1 tablespoon organic honey, and 1/10 teaspoon of cayenne pepper to 10 ounces of hot water. Cayenne pepper is used in these drinks because of its ability to increase the body's metabolic rate and increase blood circulation.[123] Jeremy Safron, founder of Loving Foods and adviser to many raw food restaurants around the United States, has promoted a product similar to the Master Cleanser as an all-day diet, consisting of 1 gallon water, ½ cup lemon juice, 1/4 teaspoon sea salt, 1/8 teaspoon vanilla, 1/4 teaspoon flax oil and either honey, dates, or maple syrup for sweetening to your own taste.[124]

Throughout Stage III, as you reintroduce a higher calorie intake, I encourage you to try and eat healthy foods, which are described in numerous publications available in any bookstore or library. As I have stated repeatedly, the *KetoFast* diet focuses only on calorie totals for weight loss, and not on any particular food group, but it would be very prudent at this time to try and refine your tastes toward foods which are healthy and low in calorie. This will enable you to help prevent heart disease and cancer as you lose weight. To this end, try to eat fresh, rather than frozen foods, and have an ample supply of fruits and vegetables. Vegetables are particularly beneficial to people on a diet because their caloric density, which measures the number of calories per volume of food, is so low. This means you can eat a greater volume of food for a given calorie level. Where meat, poultry, fish and cheese average 800-2000 calories per pound, and whole grains average 600 calories per pound, green vegetables contain only about 100 calories per pound, allowing you the ability to fill your stomach more completely while on a low-calorie diet.

I will admit that this type of recommendation is relatively new for me, since all my life, I have been a meat-and-potato proponent, not because of any medical education, but from a strictly personal taste viewpoint. I truly believed in years past that the human species had a need for meat, stemming from our carnivorous genes, which favored the digestion of energy-rich foods. As I researched the literature for the preparation of this book, however, I have been impressed by the data which many vegetarians have presented about the advantages of a meat-free diet. One book in particular which has persuaded me to make some modifications in the advice I give my medical patients is *The China Study*, by T. Colin Campbell, PhD, the director of the China-Cornell-Oxford Project, which has now completed its second phase of investigation of dietary and lifestyle factors associated with disease mortality in 170 villages in mainland China and Taiwan.[125] This study compared two populations with a similar genetic heritage, but with radically different diets. The average rural Chinese diet contains about 15% fat, while many Chinese residents in cities consume a more typical Western diet, containing about 30-45% of calories from fat, primarily animal-based. The percentage of calories from animal protein in Chinese rural intake is only 0.8%, while the American western diet typically provides 10-11% of the calories from animal protein.[126] The results of the China Study clearly indicated that the rural Chinese families had a much lower incidence of both heart disease and cancer, when compared to their genetically similar city brethren. While I am not going to suggest that you refrain from eating meat altogether, I think you would find it beneficial to concentrate on expanding your intake of vegetables, which are the primary ingredients in the recipes contained herein because of their lower calorie content. The China Study also downplays the importance of milk, but I am not in favor of that proposal. I will say, however, that if you choose to drink milk, you can reduce your intake of fat by using skim milk, which has 5% of calories derived from fat, instead of Low-Fat (35% of calories from fat), or whole milk (64% of calories from fat).[127] In addition to ingesting less fat, you will take in fewer calories since 1 cup of whole milk has 150 calories, while skim milk has 85 calories.

If you are concerned about not obtaining enough amino acids from a primarily vegetable based diet, note that the recently updated Dietary Reference

46

Intake guidelines recommend that adult women only need 46 grams of protein per day, and men 56 grams, levels that are easier to achieve than those previously recommended.[128] As a yardstick, one glass of milk contains about 8 grams of protein. Meat, milk, eggs and soy contain all the essential amino acids, while vegetables often lack certain ones, but by combining different vegetable sources in your diet, you can supply an adequate amount of all the essential amino acids throughout the course of the day. Vegetables which are particularly rich in the essential amino acids include soybeans, lentils, nuts, chickpeas, and flaxseeds.[129] Note that if you are very athletic, or have a large muscle mass, your need for protein intake rises about 50%.

VI. RULES OF THE ROAD TO WEIGHT LOSS SUCCESS

There are some easy-to-understand rules which should be followed in order to assure that your *KetoFast* program will be safe and successful. While an old adage advises that some rules are made to be broken, these rules are not. It is essential that you read this section carefully, and educate yourself to suggestions that will finally break your record of weight-loss failure.

A. Rule 1. Evaluate Your General Health

Do not begin the program until you have discussed the status of your health with your own physician. You must be sure that you have no health problems which make you more susceptible to damage from the development of slight acidosis. Conditions such as Diabetes Mellitus, Hypothyroidism, and Hypertension do not necessarily mean the diet cannot be utilized, but these disorders may require closer supervision by a physician to assure that problems do not arise. Diabetic medication, in particular, requires that you maintain a continuous intake of calories to prevent serious reactions of hypoglycemia (low blood sugar), and I do not recommend you follow this program unless you can discontinue the medication, while periodically checking your blood sugar to be sure it does not reach dangerous levels above 250. Short-term hyperglycemia, or fasting blood sugar levels above the normal of 100-110, are not dangerous, but if levels are persistently above 200, medication may have to be restarted.

Hypertension will also generally require less medication amounts during Stages I and II, but you should first ask your physician if it is safe to stop, or lower your dosage of medication while on the *KetoFast* diet. The drop in blood pressure is primarily due to a decline in sympathetic nervous activity, which is frequently increased in obesity,[130] but is also due, in part, to the associated water and sodium loss which takes place during the initial phases of fasting. If you do reduce your hypertensive medication, take your blood pressure daily at home, and notify your physician if levels consistently raise above 130/80, the upper limit of normal.

Unstable angina pectoris (heart pain), recent myocardial infarction within the past three months, malignant dysrrhythmias of the heart, such as paroxysmal ventricular tachycardia and the prolonged QT syndrome, pregnancy, severe renal (kidney) or hepatic (liver) disease, and recurrent syncope (fainting) are generally felt to be contraindications to undergoing a prolonged starvation or VLCD phase, which is part of the *KetoFast* program. In addition, recent or recurrent cerebrovascular accidents (CVAs) and/or transient ischemic attacks (TIAs) should be viewed as contraindications to utilizing this diet. If your own physician disagrees with utilizing my weight-loss methodology, I suggest you ask the reasons why, and query if the resistance is due to a general disbelief in the philosophy of water-fasts or

VLCD calorie control, or because you have some specific medical disorder which would make utilizing these methods for a short period of time dangerous. I cannot provide professional advice on your particular state of health, and it is incumbent upon you to satisfy your concerns with information provided by physicians in your area. If necessary, get a second opinion from a physician who is knowledgeable about weight-loss problems.

You should also be aware that any successful diet program is associated with an increased incidence of symptomatic cholelithiasis (gall stones), for reasons that are still unknown. If you develop pain in your abdomen, particularly in the right upper quadrant, with or without nausea, you should check with your physician and be examined.

B. Rule 2. Learn to Cook Your Own Food

It is important that you learn to cook your own food, or at least take a major part in the process, during Stage II. If you follow this program carefully, and train yourself to eat a smaller volume of properly prepared food, you will have learned a method of dieting that will last your whole life. I have explained a number of times that it is essential that you take part in the cooking process, for you must learn how to control the volume of food you eat by training yourself to understand how many calories are likely to be present on a plate of food put before you at a restaurant or your neighbor's home. You have a genetic deficiency of some type of hormonal or enzymatic pathway, and you simply cannot eat the quantity of food which normal individuals can consume. As discussed earlier, if you spill ketones within 24-48 hours of a fast, you task to lose weight is simple: **if it tastes good, spit it out.** If you don't burn fat within that period of time, you will have to learn to eat smaller portions of food than your friends, until the cause of your problem is discovered, and medication becomes available. You can only do this by gaining experience in what a 100-calorie portion looks like. Remember that 50 calories truly makes a difference with your genetic deficiency, so put on an apron and get to work.

C. Rule 3. Drink 6 Glasses of Water Each Day

It is very important that you maintain an adequate fluid intake in order to effectively wash the ketone products out of your blood and into the urinary tract as soon as your fat is catabolized. Total fluid intake should always exceed 1500-2000 ml per day (2 quarts or 4 full size water-bottles or 6-7 8-ounce glasses). Although some enthusiasts claim that dark-colored urine may occur because of toxin cleansing,[131] you should always take it to mean that you are not drinking enough water, which leads to dehydration, and a darker than normal urine color. If possible, the beverages should be cold, for it has been shown that you can burn extra calories by "water-induced thermogenesis." A group of researchers at the Charite, Humboldt-University in Berlin studied the effects of drinking 500 ml of water (17 ounces, or about one pint) on energy

50

expenditure and found that cold water increased the metabolic rate by 30%, for a total of almost 25 calories (100 kilojoules).[132] Drinking 2 liters of water a day would therefore use almost 100 calories, a significant expenditure when you are only taking in a few hundred calories at the start of Stage II. It should be noted, however, that this same amount of water ingestion can increase blood pressure in older individuals, and so you should check your blood pressure on a regular basis if you have Hypertension and plan to drink this volume of liquid daily.[133]

The fluid intake should primarily be water, but you can include diet beverages if desired. At the start of the diet, all fluids should be caffeine-free, so that you can begin your measurement of weight loss without the diuretic effect of caffeine, which will overestimate your desired goals by accelerating the loss of water. Advocates of a water-fast to promote detoxification of the body often do not allow ingestion of caffeinated beverages, claiming that the resultant stimulation of the nervous system interferes with the cleansing process, but I do not find that this precaution is necessary for weight loss, although I encourage you to keep your caffeine intake to a minimum. Caffeine is a xanthine alkaloid compound that is found in the leaves and beans of the coffee plant, as well as in tea, yerba mate, guarana berries, the kola nut, and in cocoa. Since it is a central nervous system stimulant, which wards off drowsiness and restores alertness, it also is added to a variety of beverages, and it is estimated that 90% of North American adults consume caffeine on a daily basis. Because caffeine causes a build up in the number of adenosine receptors in the brain by its daily use, you may encounter unwelcome symptoms during withdrawal, such as headache, nausea, irritability and fatigue. For this reason, I recommend that you take caffeine out of your diet for one week before beginning Stage I, as some patients experience similar symptoms during a water-fast, and you will lessen the intensity by withdrawing the caffeine first. It also will allow you to begin your diet at a baseline of water content that is not affected by the diuretic effect of caffeine. This may increase your initial loss of weight because of water-loss, but it will be part of the natural response to lowered sodium intake, rather than chemical diuresis.

Once you are in Stage II, it is generally accepted that up to 300 mg of caffeine daily (the equivalent of three cups of coffee, six to seven cups of tea, or six servings of cola drinks) is beneficial and safe, and may even increase the release of fat from adipocytes and boost the rate of fat burning, although it has not yet been shown to specifically increase the likelihood of weight loss during calorie-restricted diets. At doses above 600 mg or more per day, caffeine can cause nervousness, sweating, tenseness, upset stomach, anxiety and insomnia, so you should keep your intake to a moderate level.

For those who do not want to take caffeine directly, the South American herb guarana (*Paullinia cupana*) can be taken in doses of 100-500 mg per day, as a stimulant to ease appetite and elevate energy expenditure. Ma huang (ephedra) is a more potent stimulant in this regard, but I do not recommend its usage during periods of severe caloric restriction because of the side effects of insomnia, irritability, and heart palpitations. Green tea, because of its caffeine and polyphenol content, has also been shown to increase energy expenditure in animals and humans, and some researchers claim that it will assist weight loss through this effect, calculating that drinking 2-3 cups per day can burn as many as 90 calories.[134]

Once again, there are divergent opinions on the benefits or dangers of caffeine, and I will leave it up to you to decide whether the stimulation of the product is beneficial to your own inherent metabolism. If you feel better taking caffeine, go ahead, but make sure you do not take more than 2 cups of caffeinated coffee or tea daily.

Although it is possible that you may feel bloated by increasing the amount of water intake, and you even may feel slight swelling in your hands or feet, this is usually a temporary phenomenon, and a proper homeostasis will soon be reached. As long as the blood flow to your kidney is maintained by keeping an adequate level of hydration, any excess water will eventually be eliminated, and the feeling of bloating will pass. Some patients, however, do retain water with normal renal and cardiovascular function, and have to take diuretics ("water pills") to reduce this excess fluid. While I do not recommend you use such medicine to decrease water retention during Stage I and II, if you already are on such a program before beginning the diet, check with your physician to see if the medication can be withheld during this period of time. Water retention is generally more of a problem when there is the associated ingestion of salt in your food, and this is obviously absent in Stage I, and greatly diminished in Stage II.

D. Rule 4. Pay Attention to Ketones, Not Weight

Do not try and be a hero and lose weight too quickly: there is no prize for first place after the first lap of a long race. Your goal is to initiate a successful weight-loss process that can then be maintained by proper caloric intake management and exercise. While it is reassuring to see results on the scale every morning, right from the start, it is also possible to lose weight too rapidly, and then suffer a serious let-down as you regain some weight along the way. This is more likely to occur during Stage II, when fluid retention may reoccur as salt is reintroduced into the diet. Let the appearance of ketones in your urine indicate that you are losing adipose tissue, and not worry about day-to-day variations in your total weight.

Most patients can expect to lose from 5-10 pounds during the first week or two of fasting, depending on their level of obesity, but this is not due to catabolism alone, and includes loss of body water and protein as well. Since one pound of fat stores up to 3500 calories, and normal people will generally metabolize 1500-2000 calories a day from their BMR, a level which may be lower in you due to your genetic deficiency. you will lose roughly about 1 pound of fat every two days during starvation. After Stage II is reached, and caloric intake is started, the process will slow down, as discussed earlier. As a general guide, a 3-5 pound weight loss will take place weekly during Stage I, 2-3 pounds during stage II, and 1-2 pounds during stage III. Some patients who are morbidly obese may lose greater amounts than this, but the higher levels should only be allowed to continue if calorie intake has reached a level of 800-1000 calories per day, assuring adequate nutritional repletion.

E. Rule 5. Do Not Exercise Until You Can Control Your Calorie-Intake

Do not exercise until your level of ketones in the urine is stable, and you can judge how the physical exertion is affecting your program and your appetite. Physical exercise is a very important part of any long-term diet program, but it is best added after you have begun the diet, and learned how to control your intake of food. This is because there are two conflicting aspects of exercise which must be carefully balanced: stimulation of appetite, and stimulation of metabolism at the cellular level. While utilizing more calories during strenuous exertion is a very beneficial advantage, since it both increases fat catabolism and stimulates growth of muscle, it frequently is offset by an increase in appetite, which makes it hard to maintain the limited amount of food necessary at the start of the diet to get your burning of fat in gear. I therefore recommend that you hold off on exercising until you can control your intake of food successfully, usually after 2 weeks into Stage II.

For purposes of weight loss, aerobic exercise is preferred, and can be achieved by walking, biking, swimming, or any variety of Pilates or floor-exercises. "Aerobic" means "with oxygen," and refers to exercise which is performed at a moderate level of intensity over a prolonged period of time, keeping your heart rate at a constant level, generally in the range of 100-120 beats per minute (bpm) in middle-age adults, for a 20-30 minute period. Obviously, well-trained athletes can perform with much higher pulse rates, but for safety, you should not push yourself during dieting to these levels. Moderate weight training with dumbells or resistance equipment is considered "anaerobic" exercise, and is effective for toning your muscles and making you look more fit, but the appetite stimulus that generally accompanies weight-training can make it difficult to maintain the lower calorie intake allowed during Stage II. For this reason, I do not recommend you add weight training until Stage III. I will discuss this shortly in more detail.

F. Rule 6. Be Sure to Supplement Your Water-Fast and VLCD

Make sure you take a multivitamin supplementation each day, and use a tablet that contains trace minerals such as copper, zinc, manganese, chromium, selenium, and molybdenum. Although some physicians do not believe that supplementation is necessary during a fast because the body stores are quite adequate, I believe it is better to be safe than sorry, and find no reason to refrain from its use. I also encourage the use of potassium supplementation, since potassium loss from muscle catabolism can affect the heart. Most of the vegetables you eat will have adequate amounts of potassium to reach the recommended daily requirement of 1875-5625 mg (40-80 mEq), but in Stages I and II your volume of food ingestion is low, and I would suggest you supplement your intake with oral potassium products, which can be found over-the-counter (OTC) at most pharmacies and health food stores. You should take at least 25 mEq per day in a liquid or powder formulation. Foods rich in potassium include cantaloupe, oranges, avocado, strawberries, tomatoes, apricots, cucumber, cabbage, artichoke, beets, spinach, and cauliflower.

I also recommend that you take a calcium supplement each day, since urinary calcium excretion rises to quite high levels during fasting, and can cause a loss of as much as 1.5% of body calcium during a two-month fast.[135] This has been attributed to the onset of ketosis, which increases calcium excretion, and since you will be having intermittent ketosis throughout Stages II and III, it is prudent to add calcium supplementation, especially if you are a woman susceptible to the development of osteoporosis. If you are postmenopausal, you are probably already taking calcium, and you should continue this throughout the time you are on *KetoFast*. It is better to take a calcium tablet combined with vitamin D, at a dosage of at least 500-1000 mg of calcium per day. Some studies have also shown a drop in serum magnesium along with calcium, and while this mineral is present in most multivitamins, you may want to consider taking a supplement of 300 mg per day.

During prolonged dieting, especially when the fat content of food is kept to a minimum, it may also be advisable to supplement your intake of the essential omega-3 and omega-6 fatty acids. Originally designated as Vitamin F when they were discovered as essential nutrients in 1923, these particular fatty acids serve multiple functions to preserve good health, and cannot be constructed within the human body *de novo* from other components. They were termed as "essential" fatty acids because each was able to meet the growth requirements of rats given fat-free diets, and since that time it has been shown that they are able to relieve the worst symptoms of fatty acid deficiency in human beings. The terminology of the omega-3 fatty acids comes from the fact that the first double bond in the molecule exists as the third carbon-carbon bond from the terminal end of the carbon chain. The omega-6 terminology means that the first double bond is on the sixth carbon from the end of the fatty acid.

Supplementation with omega-3 and omega-6 fatty acids has become a popular health craze in recent years, with various authors claiming that these compounds have the ability to prevent the development of arteriosclerosis. This assertion has not been proven by controlled studies, but the data was impressive enough for the U.S. Food and Drug Administration (FDA) to give two of the omega-3 fatty acids, eicosapentaenoic acid (EPA) and docosahexaenoic acid (DHA), a "qualified health claim" status in 2006, by stating that "supportive but not conclusive research shows that consumption of EPA and DHA omega-3 fatty acids may reduce the risk of coronary heart disease."[136] The "supportive" and "may" components of this summary continue to leave the issue open to question, but many companies have jumped on the chance to promote the sale of these products, often at inflated prices, as a health additive. There are few detrimental side effects to taking these supplements, and since your intake of food is very limited in Stages I and II, I think it is reasonable to take some form of omega-3 at a dosage of 500-1000 mg per day.

While it has also been claimed that conjugated linoleic acid (CLA) will accelerate the burning of fat in dosages of 1-3 grams per day, the data is still inconclusive, as is the case with another omega-6 compound, gamma-linolenic acid (GLA), which is prevalent in Evening Primrose Oil (EPO), I do not believe that the data is clear enough to utilize either of these compounds as a weight-loss aid, but it would be reasonable during Stage III that you try to eat foods which provide the largest content of these essential substances, such as fish and shellfish (especially cold water oily fish such as salmon, herring, mackerel, anchovies, and sardines), flaxseed (55% ALA), hemp oil, soy beans, tofu, canola (rapeseed) oil, chia seeds (64% ALA), pumpkin seeds, sunflower seeds, leafy vegetables, and walnuts. You can also mix 1 tablespoon of flaxseed oil with ½ cup of low fat cottage cheese and have an excellent source of these important fatty acids, but remember that this will count as 200 calories towards your day's total intake, a burden when you are in Stage II, but less of a problem in Stage III.[137]

Other supplements which are sometimes recommended to patients undergoing weight loss include:

* Carnitine (L-carnitine), an amino acid that is synthesized in the liver and kidneys from lysine and methionine, which facilitates the transport and metabolism of long-chain fatty acids into the mitochondria for energy generation. This has prompted its use as an ergogenic aid, but the results have been equivocal. Patients on VLCDs have been shown to have lower levels of carnitine in the blood and tissues, prompting its use as a supplement in doses of 2-4 grams per day, but studies have failed to show significant increased weight

loss.[138] It is particularly found in red meats, so if you are a strict vegetarian, you may wish to supplement your diet with 500-1000 mgs per day. It should not be taken by people with bipolar disease or epilepsy, so you should check with your physician before utilizing this product.

* Hydroxycitric acid (HCA), which is made from the Carcinia cambogia fruit, commonly known as Malabar tamarind. It is claimed to reduce appetite, making hunger less of a problem during dieting, but strictly controlled studies have not been performed. Dried pieces of the rind of this fruit are added to curry powder in the cuisines from India, Laos, Malaysia, and Burma, but there are also extract capsules which can be taken three times a day before meals.

* Pyruvate, the anionic form of pyruvic acid, a by-product of sugar metabolism, is widely present in fruits and vegetables, as well as dark beer and red wine, and some research has suggested that it can aid in weight loss if taken in dosages of 30 grams per day. It is not clear why taking such supraphysiological levels of pyruvate may lead to fat loss, although it has been suggested that it may enhance fat oxidation.[139] Since there is still little known about the effects of this substance, I do not recommend that you take this large 30 gram dosage, but if you believe in the benefits of pyruvate, then take 5-6 grams per day in powder form, or 1-2 grams per day in tablets, recognizing the possibility that it may create some degree of abdominal bloating, gas or diarrhea.[140] Pyruvate does not come cheap, however, so be prepared to pay a hefty cost for the uncertain benefit.

* Coenzyme Q10 (ubiquinone), an antioxidant/anti-inflammatory agent, has been touted as a beneficial supplement to patients over the age of 40, aiding in the treatment of metabolic disorders, mitochondrial disorders, brain health, and Hypertension. It is often taken in doses of 30-100 mg per day, but I do not feel that it has any value in weight loss. Like many of the other OTC health products, it is quite expensive, so judge for yourself if you need to fortify your diet with this additive.

* Apple Cider Vinegar has been promoted as an aid to weight loss, as well as a cure for a variety of medical ailments. A number of products are on sale which combine apple cider vinegar with other supplements, but I do not feel they add any benefit to patients attempting to lose weight. I would not utilize it in Stage I, when all taste sensation is eliminated, but during Stages II and III, this product offers a tasty alternative to water alone, without adding many calories. Taking 2 teaspoons of apple cider vinegar in a glass of water contains only 30 calories, and provides beneficial electrolyte and malic acid content, so a daily consumption would be acceptable.

* At this time, I do not recommend taking banaba leaf, bladderwrack, chitosan, glucomannan, *Gymnema sylvestre*, Quercetin, white willow bark

(salicin), or hydroxycitric acid (HCA)(*Garcinia cambogia*). These products have been claimed to aid in weight loss by various manufacturers, but their support is simply too sparse to take as a supplement at this time.

Finally, do not take thyroid supplementation beyond your normal needs during this diet, even if you have been recommended to do so by diet doctors who have promoted taking thyroid in the form of T3 (triiodothyronine), in order to accentuate weight loss and correct the drop in serum levels of free T3, which are known to occur with dietary weight loss. While it is true that there is a drop in the level of free T3 in the blood when you lose weight, this does not mean that you are thyroid deficient, and you should not attempt to correct the problem with a prescription that will offset your normal thyroid balance. Patients who are obese have a BMR that is already 20-50% above the ideal level, and taking excess thyroid will accentuate this problem. While hyperthyroid patients may lose weight, they do it at the expense of overstimulating their cardiovascular system. I do not recommend that you resort to these techniques, even if they were to slightly increase your weight loss.

G. Rule 7. Do Not Follow *KetoFast* if You are Pregnant or Breast-Feeding

If you are a menstruating female of child-bearing age, do not follow this diet unless you are first certain you are not pregnant. Because obesity is occasionally associated with amenorrhea or delayed menstrual periods, you may not have menstrual periods every month, but do not rely on this fact to begin the diet without checking a urine pregnancy test. These are readily available, and you should always check to be sure you are not pregnant before beginning any type of restricted diet to lose weight. Most physicians recommend that during pregnancy, you not only refrain from dieting, but increase your intake of food by 150 calories per day for the first trimester, and 300 calories per day for the remainder of the pregnancy. If you are postpartum, and breast feeding, you should also should increase your intake by 500 calories per day. You may want to return to your pre-pregnancy weight as soon as possible, but do not do it at the expense of your health, and that of your baby, so wait until you wean off breast-feeding before beginning *KetoFast*.

H. Rule 8. Practice Dermal Dry Brush Exfoliation Daily

Give your skin a dry brush exfoliation every day while you are in Stage I of the diet, and follow it up with a shower to wash away the dead skin particles that have been removed by the brushing. The skin is your body's largest organ for elimination of toxins, and holistic and alternative medicine practitioners often recommend this cleansing method as a way of purging the body of deleterious products, pointing out that more than one pound of waste is excreted through the skin each day, including heavy metal compounds that are common contaminants in both the air we breathe, and the food we eat. By brushing your entire body, you remove the outer layer of dead epidermal cells, and open the pores of the skin, allowing for an uninterrupted excretory process. While I do not subscribe to the expansive claims made by many alternative-health enthusiasts, I do believe that dry brush exfoliation is beneficial to the health of your skin, and the relaxation associated with the technique is also a comforting side-effect. During Stage II, when ketosis is only intermittent, you can continue the process daily, but 1-2 times per week should provide satisfactory benefits.

The procedure is quite simple, and you can spend as much, or as little, time as you want in performing the brush massage. Be sure to purchase a natural bristle brush (plant fiber or boar bristle), rather than one made from nylon or synthetic fibers, and always employ the process before showering, as this will enable you to wash the dead epidermal cells away. Begin at your feet and move up to your torso, and then from your fingertips to the armpits, always brushing towards the heart, along the natural flow of the lymph vessels which lie below the skin. In this manner, you are not only cleansing the skin, but you are accentuating the flow of lymph fluid, which is not only involved with removing excess fluids from body tissues, aiding in the transport of fat to the circulatory system, but also aids in the production of immune cells which fight infection. The lymphatic system does not have a central pumping system like the blood, and depends on the movement of skeletal muscles to move the fluid towards the heart. Brushing assists movement of lymph during the period of time your exercise level is reduced. Do not brush any area that is irritated, or has open sores.

In addition to a dry brush process, you can take a bath using ½ cup of baking soda or Epsom salts once or twice a week to assist in the cleansing process. Make sure the water is warm, and stay in the bath for 10-20 minutes. When you are done, take a quick shower to eliminate contaminants that were dispersed in the bath water. Although some purists suggest that you only use filtered water during your bathing to prevent the absorption of chlorine through your skin, I do not believe this added expense is necessary.

I. Rule 9. Refrain from Drinking Non-Diet Beverages

Do not drink alcoholic beverages, non-diet soft drinks, or undiluted fruit juice in Stage I and II, because their calorie content will push you over your allotted limit. One bottle of beer averages 150 calories, and one bottle of light beer averages 100 calories. One jigger of Gin or Vodka averages 100 calories. One glass of table wine (3.5 fluid ounces) averages 75 calories. Root Beer, Cola, and 7-UP drinks average 150 calories per 12 fluid ounce. Undiluted fruit juices will average about 100 calories per glass. It is therefore imperative that during Stages I and II you get used to diet-drinks or water, or dilute your fruit juice at least threefold. Once you enter Stage III, you can once again begin to imbibe your choice of alcoholic beverage, but remember to take note of the calorie load and drink in moderation. While all "beer-bellies" are not from the effects of alcohol alone, it is unlikely that they will be reduced without some attempt at temperance. Unsweetened coffee or tea are acceptable alternatives.

In addition to limiting the alcohol and calorie content of your drinks, you should try and keep carbonation to a minimum. Liquids are carbonated by impregnation with carbon dioxide (CO_2), and while there is no evidence that the chemical itself is dangerous, the bubbles which are produced can induce the stomach to secrete more gastric acid. Under normal dietary conditions, this acidity is neutralized quickly by the food you eat, but in Stage I and II, when there is little calorie intake, you are in danger of developing gastritis, leading to pain and nausea. The increase in gastric acid secretion is compounded by the fact that carbon dioxide reacts with water (H_2O) to form carbonic acid ($H2CO_3$). When the stomach is dilated by the gaseous discharge (an 8-ounce glass of carbonated beverage distends the stomach 16 ounces), there is reflux of acid from the stomach into the esophagus, which also increases the complaint of heartburn.

VII. DETAILED INSTRUCTION OF THE *KETOFAST* DIET PROGRAM

See, that wasn't so bad, was it? A few rules and you're set to go. There is very little equipment that you will have to buy in order to follow this diet, but a few things are essential. First, although you will not need a "calorie counter" during Stages I and II if you plan to only follow the recipes in this book, I highly suggest you buy one now and utilize it whenever possible to learn how many calories are in the foods you like to eat. Eventually, you will want to modify your intake to fit your personal tastes, and it will then be necessary to calculate the caloric intake of what you eat. An important part of this process involves paying attention to the small portions by which each food's calorie content is determined. If your calorie-counter says that a 3-ounce portion of fish has 100 calories, you cannot eat 6 ounces and expect to moderate your calorie intake enough to allow for catabolism of fat. Since you suffer from a genetic deficiency of some type of weight control hormone or enzymatic pathway, a 100 calorie difference can turn off your pilot light of fat catabolism.

The *KetoFast* diet does not differentiate the source of the calorie, be it protein, carbohydrate, or fat. What matters most is the total number of calories you eat. You may have encountered some diets which stress a particular food group and tell you to avoid certain others. I do not believe that any food substance is more important than any other for the purposes of weight loss. Although other health factors may determine whether you should eat less fat or protein, for right now it is the calorie intake itself that determines whether you will lose weight or not. Exact accuracy of measuring calorie intake is not critical in the maintenance phase of the program, but in Stage II it is essential that you not exceed 600 calories a day in order to begin proper burning of fat cells.

You will need a supply of urine test tapes to measure the amount of ketone in the urine. These are available at most drugstores, and also can be purchased online from many sources. They are reasonably priced, and are an essential part of your ability to monitor your progress throughout Stages II and III. The only other piece of equipment is a scale. This does not have to be expensive, or even accurate, for it is the change from day-to-day that is more important than the accuracy of the weight itself. You may even elect to do what my wife once did when we moved into a new home: step on every scale in the store and buy the one that shows the lowest weight. As I said, if the scale you bring home reflects that you are losing weight, it does not matter whether the total amount is accurate, when compared to expensive scales in physician offices. In order to follow your progress, weigh yourself at the start of the diet, and then continue to check your weight every morning, keeping a record of each result in order to follow your progress. Do not be disturbed if your weight does not decrease daily, as fluctuations of weight due to varying degrees of water retention are to be expected. Pay more attention to what you lose on a weekly basis, but take the weight daily in order to have a more accurate series of weights to graph your response.

OK, you're ready to start, let's go.

A. Stage I

This is where the program of dietary education to help you lose weight for the rest of your life begins. You are reading this book because your physiologic pilot light, which is responsible for the burning of fat during periods of caloric restriction, cannot be properly maintained during a normal intake of food. You lack a hormone that instructs your body to burn fat at appropriate intervals, or an enzymatic pathway that enables proper catabolism to take place, and as a result you have gained weight at calorie intake levels that would not cause a similar problem in other individuals. In order to modify your system, and achieve a more normal response to caloric restriction, you have to "start the fires burning" by initiating a carefully monitored zero-caloric water fast, and begin to live off the fat of your own land.

An understanding of the rate at which your are burning your fat cells in Stage I will help you progress once you enter Stage II. First, make a recording sheet in order to keep a record of your output of ketones in the urine. You can simply make 5 columns on a sheet of paper, with the first column being the date and time you test your urine, and the next 4 columns the results. You will be measuring the amount of ketone in the urine four times daily. The first urine specimen is taken immediately upon awakening in the morning. Because your urine at that time will consist of substances excreted by the kidney throughout the nighttime hours, it will give you an accurate indication of whether fat cells were catabolized throughout the evening hours while you slept. The specimens which follow will tell you whether fat catabolism is turned on or off.

During Stage I, when ketone output will reach the highest levels possible, it is imperative that you drink at least six 8-ounce glasses of water, or some form of sugar-free beverage, each day. Your liquids must be sugar-free, since 5 teaspoons of sugar contain 100 calories. The total fluid intake should be over 1500 ml (50 ounces, 1 ½ quarts, 6 8-ounce glasses), so that you can adequately flush your system of circulating ketones, and maintain a good urine flow to aid in the testing process. Many alternative health practitioners demand that you drink only distilled (chemical and mineral free) or purified water, rather than chlorinated tap water, which became standard in water treatment across the country in 1904. Chlorine can combine with organic materials to form trihalomethanes (THMs), which are highly carcinogenic. Although some scientists claim that drinking tap water can increase your rate of developing bladder and rectal cancer by 93%, pointing to a report by the U. S. Council of Environmental Quality (CEQ),[141] most researchers believe that the danger is minimal, and that tap water is safe to drink. I will leave this decision up to you, since attempting to refrain from standard water sources requires a long-term commitment that you may or may not be willing to make. I would point out that it is not only more costly to purchase large amounts of purified water, but it adds a significant burden of container recycling on the environment, as there are now 22 billion water bottles thrown away each year, taking as long as 1,000 years to biodegrade. In addition, recent data indicates that many of the plastic bottles can contaminate the water you drink with chemical carcinogens, such as Bisphenol A (BPA) and di(2-ethylhexyl) phthalate (DEHP). If you are serious about purifying your water source, consider buying a home water-purifier rather than relying on these external sources.

Because you are drinking more water than you may have been before, it is likely that you will be urinating more frequently, and it should be easy to obtain a specimen of urine, even if you have recently emptied your bladder. If you find that it takes longer than expected to obtain a urine specimen, increase your fluid intake so that the rate of urine flow is stimulated. If you choose to have flavored liquids rather than water, avoid carbonated drinks. Ingested gas can stimulate gastric acid secretion, and since you are not eating any food during Stage I, you will not be able to buffer the acid, possibly leading to mild gastritis (stomach inflammation) and acid indigestion. Taking some type of antacid on a regular basis during these first few days, such as TUMS or Mylanta, may be beneficial, especially if you choose to take carbonation. Caffeine is also an acid stimulant, so you should avoid beverages with caffeine and have only the decaffeinated variety during Stage I.

Measurements of the urine should be taken four times daily: immediately before breakfast, lunch, dinner, and bedtime. Since you are not actually eating during Stage I, the exact timing is not important, but for consistency with later measurements, I recommend that you test the urine just before meals would normally be taken. In this way, you will begin to learn a pattern that will become more comfortable as time goes by. If you get up in the middle of the night to urinate (nocturia), it is not necessary to test your urine, although if this becomes a nightly occurrence you may wish to have your urine tested for the presence of glucose (glucosuria), just to be sure you are not showing signs of uncontrolled Diabetes Mellitus. Ketostix strips do not denote the presence of glucose, and you will have to either see your physician, or borrow a glucose test-strip from a friend with Diabetes. *KetoFast* does not cause Diabetes Mellitus, and will actually improve the disease in the long-run, but you should still be careful to be aware of the cause of your nocturia, and whether your obesity has finally led to a diabetic condition. The more understanding you can have of the way your body reacts to calorie restriction, the better you will be able to determine how long it will be necessary to maintain these dietary requirements.

Whether you elect to sit at the table with the rest of the family during meal times, or remain at a distance because of the strong appeal of food, is a personal decision. Just as some people who stop smoking cannot be exposed to the smell of smoke, or alcoholics who go through withdrawal cannot return to socialize at places where their friends continue to drink alcohol, you have to determine how well you can handle the sight and smell of food while undergoing this period of water-fasting, especially at the start of the program. Learning self-control over the urges of appetite early on is beneficial to your eventual goal of weight control, but some people simply cannot deal with the stimulation to eat that accompanies the sight and smell of food. Do not worry that this is a sign of weakness. As you develop mild ketosis, your appetite will diminish, and it is probable that you will be able to change your habits as soon as the process has reached Stage II.

Testing the urine for ketones is so easy that anyone could become proficient at once. The actual insertion of the test-strip into the urine specimen can be carried out in one of two ways. The easiest method is to hold the dipstick directly in the urine stream, without diversion into a separate receptacle. It is possible, however, that some spraying of urine will result, which will require a cleansing of the affected area. Although few urine specimens actually contain infectious material, good cleansing procedures are still recommended when there is contamination by urine. Many people choose to urinate into a cup, and then dip the strip into the urine and test for ketones before disposing of the urine into the toilet. The cup does not have to be sterile, but should be rinsed out before reuse. Either method is satisfactory for the purposes at hand, but the test-strip must be thoroughly wetted to assure an accurate reading. Very little urine is needed to accomplish this task, and there are few substances which will give a false reading.

Instructions on how to read the test-strip to quantitate the amount of ketone in the urine will depend on the particular product you are using. All methods, however, work on the same general principle. The most popular product, "Ketostix," has a chemical reagent imbedded on one end of the strip, usually sodium nitroprusside, that will react with ketones in the urine to provide a color change.[142] The color produced will be dependent on the amount of ketones present, and a color chart on the bottle allows you to determine the concentration of ketones. There will also be directions on how long to wait before reading the color change, typically fifteen seconds. The values of ketone concentration will generally be listed as none, trace (5 mg/dl), small (15 mg/dl), moderate (40mg/dl), and large (160 mg/dl), and this is the value you are to record in your chart for compilation. Other ketone test-strips which are readily available at drugstores and on the Internet include "ReliOn," "Ketone generic test strips," "Ketogenic," and "LWS ketone strips."

As a summary, there will be three steps:

1. Remove one strip from the bottle and dip the test area in the urine or urine stream. Make sure you totally immerse the specified section.
2. Wait the required period of time for a color change to occur.
3. Compare the color change on the test-strip with the color chart on the container and record the result on your daily record.

This is so simple that you can do it in any washroom facility without attracting undue attention. The test-strip may float on top of the water in the toilet bowl, so it is preferable to discard it into a waste receptacle if you are using a public washroom. The whole process will take less than one minute, repeated four times a day, and in those four minutes you will obtain an enormous amount of information on the status of your fat metabolism. Since the production of ketones in the body is reflected by the excretion of ketones in the urine, you can use this measurement as an index of how much fat catabolism is taking place throughout your body. When there are no ketones present, there is no utilization of fat as an energy source. Your system is using glucose that has been recently consumed, or converted from glycogen stores or protein. As the amount of ketones in the urine rises, you are beginning to utilize mobilized fatty acids that have come from triglyceride sources in your adipose tissue. This means that your pilot light of fat catabolism has been lit, and you are burning fat at an acceptable rate.

As you are checking your weight every morning on the scale when you first wake up, remember that some reduction is going to occur before fat is actually being burned. This is due to the loss of water which was discussed earlier, and eventually this loss will be restored, once the body senses a reduction in blood volume. Because this is likely to occur as fat loss begins, the level of your weight will appear to plateau as the two cancel each other out. Burning of fat will push the weight lower, but reaccumulation of water will edge it upward. This is not a sign that the diet is failing, so remember to pay less attention to the level of your weight at this point, and believe more in the measurement of urine ketones, which will give you a more accurate reflection of actual fat loss. If the urine test is positive for ketones, you are burning fat and the level of your weight is immaterial.

Your stomach will be prone to developing gastritis from medications which have an irritative effect on the mucosal lining, so if you develop pain for any reason, you should only take acetaminophen (Tylenol), and refrain from the intake of aspirin, naproxyn (Alleve), or ibuprofen (Advil, Motrin) until you begin to ingest more than 1000 calories a day. Occasionally stomach acid output is great enough to cause symptoms of indigestion even when stimulants, or irritative compounds are not ingested. Under these circumstances, you should take OTC preparations such as liquid antacids or Zantac, Tagamet, or Pepcid AC. In order to reduce the output of acid, do not chew gum, as this is a stimulant for the secretion of digestive juices.

Because you are only taking liquids during this initial phase of the diet, and are not ingesting the recommended amounts of dietary fiber that make up a healthy menu, you may encounter a mild amount of constipation, especially if you are on medications which have this condition as a side-effect. Drugs such as calcium-channel blockers for Hypertension, anti-depressants, iron pills, and pain pills frequently cause mild constipation, and their potency in this regard may be stimulated by the dietary changes of calorie-restriction. In the VLCDs utilized by the Apfelbaums in Paris, France, patients averaged only two bowel movements per week,[143] and although this is not a dangerous problem, if you are concerned that your system has had problems of this type before, you can supplement your water-fast with both stool softeners, and sugar-free fiber products.

Stool softeners, such as Colace (Purdue Pharma, L.P.), are encapsulated oils (docusate) that can be taken once or twice daily to help prevent dehydration of the feces from creating a hard stool which will be difficult to pass. They have few side effects, and are easy to take, although with long-term use they can affect the absorption of certain nutrients. Fiber products are undigestable fibers that swell when combined with water in the stomach, adding bulk to the stool and allowing for a suitable bowel movement, since stimulation to eliminate is more likely to occur when the stool is large enough to dilate the rectum. Fibers are found primarily in wheat products, vegetables, beans, oats, and fruit skins, and can either be water-insoluble fibers, such as the skin of fruit and potatoes, wheat and corn bran, flax seed, and vegetables like celery and green beans, or water-soluble fibers, such as the pulp of fruits, and edible parts of plants. Horace Fletcher (1849-1919), the early twentieth century self-proclaimed health-food fadist, nicknamed the "Great Masticator," once advised patients to chew each mouthful of food at least 32 times before swallowing, and then spit out the remaining fiber content as you would a cherry pit. He argued that this technique, known as "Fletcherizing," would turn a "pitiable glutton into an intelligent epicurean," by eliminating the non-nutritious fiber component of food.[144] His advice is ridiculed today, and maintaining a proper intake of fiber is felt to be an essential component of maintaining healthy gastrointestinal function and preventing colon cancer.

OTC fiber preparations are available if you are averse to eating fiber, or are on a prolonged juice-diet. They are usually in powder form, which are mixed with water and taken once or twice daily, and include products like Citrucel (GlaxoSmithKline) and Celevac (Shire), made from methycelllulose, and Metamucil (Proctor & Gamble), which contains psyllium seed husks. As an alternative, you can take 1 teaspoon of psyllium husk powder in 2-4 ounces of water. Let your taste buds and pocketbook help you decide what product to use, since palatability is an issue with some people.

Practitioners of juice-fasts often take 1-2 tablespoon of ground flax seeds in a glass of water once or twice daily to prevent constipation, but remember that 2 tablespoons of flaxseeds adds 85 calories to your intake. Flax seeds can also be sprinkled over your meals if you do not like the taste or consistency in water. If constipation is still a problem, you can try herbal laxative teas, made from senna leaf, which are readily available at many health-food stores, taken at bedtime. Another option is to drink a salt water solution known as "internal salt water bathing," which flushes the colon without resorting to an enema. It is prepared by mixing 1-quart of warm distilled or purified water (1.5 liter, 2.7 fluid ounces) with two level teaspoons of non-iodized sea salt (not ordinary table salt), and then ingesting it first thing in the morning on an empty stomach.[145] You should not take any supplements or food, except for water, until the salt water is out of your stomach (about 2 hours). Because the response is unpredictable, I suggest that you only take ½ quart the first time you try this approach.

Dr. Otto Buchinger, Sr. (1876-1966), who championed the use of juice-fasts in Germany in the 1920s, and is said to have supervised over 100,000 juice-fasting cures, utilized a product known as Glauber's salts (sodium sulfate), named after Johann Rudolf Glauber, who discovered the salt crystals in Hungarian spring water in the 17th century. Buchinger dissolved 1 ½ ounces of the salts in 1 1/4 pints of warm water, and had his patients take it on the first day of fasting with a glass of fruit juice to modify the taste.[146] N. W. Walker (1866-1984), D. Sc., who championed the use of raw vegetables and juices, also used Glauber salts, which was bottled in French Lick, Indiana as Pluto Water in the early twentieth century.[147] Some European Clinics use Castor oil for the same purpose. I do not believe that the individual product is important, but some type of encouragement of bowel movements on an every 1-3 day basis is certainly a good idea.

Although alternative-medicine advocates frequently recommend the use of enemas during periods of fast to help remove toxins from the colon, claiming that such a technique removes "years of accumulated debris and mucus,"[148] I do not believe that you should do this on a regular basis. Herbert Shelton, who directed more water-fasts than anyone else in this country, also was against the use of enemas, claiming that daily enemas were not only unnecessary, "they are actually hurtful."[149] Stagnated stool does indeed remain in the colon for days before it is totally eliminated, but the use of a flow enema, rather than a cathartic, can induce bacteremia by forcing the bacteria into the blood stream through the pliable intestinal wall. If you are uncomfortable from the reduced amount of bowel movement, I would recommend that you take an OTC glycerin suppository, although an occasional enema would not be detrimental, as long as you do not do this on a daily basis. If you do believe in the advantages of enemas during periods of fasting, I suggest that you only take 1 quart of lukewarm water with a few drops of lemon juice added, or 1 tablespoon of sea salt or Vinegar, and not attempt to undergo full colonic cleansings, which require the assistance of an experienced practitioner. Be sure to use some type of lubricant on the speculum, such as Vaseline or KY Jelly, before inserting into the rectum. Try to retain the enema solution for 5-15 minutes before expulsion. Never share the enema with other users, even if you cleanse the components. The cost savings is not worth the risk of insufficient sterilization.

If you do not want to take anything to assist you in having a bowel movement when you enter Stage II, try to pick foods with high fiber content as soon as possible. In order to assure that the fibers will swell to a proper size, be sure to drink the allotted 6-8 glasses of water a day, which will assist elimination from both the kidney and GI tract. I will highlight some recipes for these products at the end of the book.

As I cautioned above, do not exercise during Stage I, and for 2 weeks in Stage II, despite the fact that popular figures like Mahatma Gandhi (1869-1948) and Dick Gregory, as well as a multitude of other people who have fasted for religious or social reasons, have shown that you can tolerate much exercise during a prolonged fast, once you are a practiced advocate. Gandhi was one of the first fasters who walked extensively during his fasts, consuming only water with citrons and honey, and popularizing a technique which spread throughout Europe. In 1954 and 1965, "fast marches" took place in Sweden with participants walking from Gothenburg to Stockholm, a distance of over 325 miles, in 10 days while ingesting only water. These adherents had spent years becoing expert in the technique, however, and neophytes should refrain from such expenditures of energy. At many of the fasting spas in Europe, it is mandatory that you rest in bed between noon and 3 PM, with hot-water bottle liver packs applied to the skin over the liver to increase circulation and assist in detoxification.[150] I do not believe you need to modify your daily activities in this manner, but I do suggest you refrain from exercise during Stage I, and early Stage II.

Since blood pressure frequently drops during Stage I, at times quite dramatically, you should discuss with your physician about decreasing medication for Hypertension before you embark on the water-fast. You should also check your blood pressure a few times each day if you have Hypertension, in order to monitor excessive fluctuations. The blood pressure may especially drop when you suddenly stand (orthostatic hypotension) or urinate, so men are advised to sit when they urinate, and both men and women should take care when rising in the morning. It is best to first sit in bed for a minute, and then stand slowly. If you do feel lightheaded, lie back down and elevate your legs. This drop in blood pressure is accentuated by dehydration, so be sure to maintain an adequate fluid intake if you remain on medication. If your blood pressure falls to systolic levels below 100, stop the water-fast and consult with your doctor about possible causes which may be undiagnosed before continuing further.

Some patients may experience vomiting the first few days of a water-fast, a side-effect blamed on the elimination of toxins by some practitioners. This explanation is not acceptable, in my opinion, and more likely indicates an underlying inflammation of the stomach (gastritis), due either to medications such as aspirin, Advil, or Alleve, or to undiagnosed gastro-esophageal reflux disease (GERD). When you cease eating food, you eliminate the buffering of stomach acidity, and may exacerbate the intensity of a subclinical underlying problem. I therefore recommend that you seek medical attention if vomiting takes place before continuing with the water-fast, and not follow the advice of alternate-health practitioners that you continue the fast and wait for the vomiting to resolve.

You may also suffer an initial exacerbation of headaches during the first few days of a water-fast, especially if you have been drinking significant amounts of caffeinated beverages, such as coffee, tea or soft drinks. This problem will usually resolve without medical attention, but remember to use only Tylenol for pain relief during Stage I, as the other medications are likely to inflame the stomach further, and lead to symptoms of gastritis. Once you begin to develop ketonuria and enter Stage II of the diet, you are likely to undergo an improvement in your headache frequency if you suffer from chronic headaches, since eating fewer calories will automatically reduce your intake of foods which can exacerbate the onset of headache in certain patients. While headaches do not require immediate attention, if they persist for more than 1-2 days, do not accept that the cause is the water-fast, and call your physician for advice.

I do not generally advise that anyone remain on a zero-calorie fast for more than 10 days, as this length of time has been shown to be safe in many studies. The popular Bragg fasting program, expounded by Paul C. Bragg

(1895-1976), who refers to himself as a "life extension specialist," calls for four 7-10 day fasts four times a year, with 24-hour fasts in between.[151] In Germany, fasting resorts typically continue the program for 21 days, while in England a 30-day fast is felt to be ideal. This length of time, however, should be reserved for those who have practiced fasting under professional guidance before, and shown themselves to be able to tolerate the treatment well. Neophytes should restrict themselves to less than 10 days.

If you have your blood tested during the initial water-fast stage, do not be concerned if cholesterol and triglyceride levels initially rise, for when fats are being broken down in the tissues and excreted into the blood as an energy source, their levels in the blood may temporarily elevate. While there has been no evidence that strokes or heart attacks are precipitated by this rise in lipid level, it is better to keep your results as low as possible after you begin the fasting stage, so that the elevations can be moderated. I therefore recommend that you hold the medication during Stage I, when no food is taken, but restart it with your first meal in Stage II. Do not decrease the amount of lipid-lowering medication you take until you have lost 10% of your body weight. With time, your levels of cholesterol and triglycerides will most likely be able to be normalized without the use of medication.

B. Stage II

Once you have reached Stage II, you have finally shifted your body metabolism into a fat-burning mode, and you are well on your way to being able to control weight gain for the rest of your life. You must now learn to monitor the process of fat catabolism by measuring the output of ketones in your urine as you slowly add 100-calorie increments. In this way, you assure that ketone production remains present, and burning of adipose tissue continues at an adequate level.

There are two important phases that you will pass through in Stage II. Phase One takes you up to 600 calories per day, and Phase Two introduces exercise and slowly increases your calorie intake to 1000 calories per day. Although I have picked 600 calories as the optimum level of intake during Phase One, if you find that you are comfortable at 500 calories, it is safe to remain at this level of intake for at least 2-3 months.

1. Phase One

Phase One begins once you have achieved an output of ketones in the urine that shows moderate or large readings on two consecutive specimens while in the water-fasting phase. It is important that the readings truly represent significant amounts of ketone production, and not be secondary to dehydrated specimens that have only concentrated ketones so that they appear to be more prominent. For this reason, do not begin Phase One until you are assured that your intake of fluids has properly diluted your urine output.

Since studies of patients on VLCDs have shown a 10-fold elevation of serum b-hydroxybutyrate, whether the diet was a Cambridge or pure-protein diet, it is possible that you may continue to show ketone production even when ingesting 600 calories a day.[152] This does not mean that every urine specimen will show the presence of ketones, but many of the specimens may be positive, as long as your 100-calorie portions of food are accurate. Previous published studies on VLCDs did not test to see if any of the patients fit your category of genetic deficiency as defined by delayed ketone production, however, so it is possible that your ketone production will shut off at lower totals than were seen with the artificial diets. For this reason, you must continue to test your metabolic system by measuring your urine ketones 4 times daily as you proceed through Phase One.

Begin caloric intake by first taking a 100-calorie portion in the evening for dinner, as this will not stimulate significant insulin excretion, which is most intense in the morning. The pancreas secretes less insulin at night, allowing for the maintenance of adequate blood glucose levels when you sleep, leading to the French proverb *Qui dort, dine*, or "sleeping is dining."[153] Taking your first meal at dinnertime also will enable you to restart medication for Hypercholesterolemia, which typically is taken with the evening meal. Do this for 2 days, and then add another 100-calorie portion for lunch on the third day. Maintain the 200 calorie total for another two days, and on the fifth day take three 100-calorie portions, one for breakfast, lunch, and dinner. If you continue to show at least one urine with ketones present, maintain this intake for two more days. As long as there is some ketone output, go to 400 calories on the seventh day, divided into 4 portions: breakfast, lunch, dinner, and bedtime. Continue this intake for 7 more days before attempting to increase to the 500 calorie level. If you do not show at least one ketone positive urine throughout the day, remain at 400 calories for another week. As I will discuss shortly, researchers have found that a 400-600 calorie diet can be safely taken for 2 months, so if your hormonal or enzymatic deficiency is severe, you need not worry that your intake is severely limited for that length of time. Since you are weighing yourself daily, you can easily determine if weight loss is taking place. If it is, do not worry about the ketone output, as you are burning fat at this stage and not losing water. If your weight remains stable for over 3 days, and your urine still does not show the presence of ketones, reduce your intake by 100 calories until ketones once again appear. If you continue to spill ketones at 500 calories, increase your total to 600 calories per day, and once again watch for the presence of fat catabolism by either weight loss or the occasional presence of ketones in the urine.

Be aware that hunger may become more of a problem during Phase One than it was during the zero-calorie fast. Once you begin to eat small amounts of food, the anticipation of eating is heightened, and the gastric juices begin to flow in response to their digestive stimulation. The ability to maintain a small ketone excretion, however, aids in controlling the degree of this appetite resurgence, making it easier to follow a 600 calorie diet, than it would to follow one of 1000 calories. As you see the pounds fall off your body, you also will be reinforced to maintain your limited intake, although control will once again be more of a problem in Stage III and beyond.

Constipation may also continue to be a problem throughout this phase, and adding fiber in the food you consume is very beneficial. One obvious choice is to use raw vegetables in the form of a salad, which is socially well-accepted as a full meal. You may buy low-calorie dressings that are commercially available (below 20 calories per 2 tablespoons), or prepare your own dressings to match your particular tastes, using sugar-free substitutes and minimum amounts of an oil base. You also can utilize some of the dressings which appear in the recipe section of this book. Many people carry a small container of these homemade dressings to restaurants so that they can order their salads dry and add the seasoning on their own. Balsamic vinegar by itself is an optimum dressing, since it has only 10 calories per tablespoon, but many people find the taste too tart. Lemon juice by itself is also a low-cal alternative. Oil, although it is good for keeping the stool soft, does have caloric content and must be added to the tabulation when you total your calorie intake for a salad. One teaspoon of olive oil has 40 calories, even though its fat content is generally considered to be healthy. It is very important that you familiarize yourself with the calorie intake of the vegetables you ingest, not only by the type of food you eat, but by the volume as well. Remember that almost every food will have some calorie content, even if it is in the form of a salad.

Most people will find that they can move up to 600 calories per day without any significant problems of losing occasional ketone excretion. Every so often, an individual will actually stop burning fat at under 500 calories a day, as was described earlier in the patient I had admitted to the hospital for gall-bladder surgery, but this is rare. If it should happen to you, first carefully check your intake of calories and be sure you are not exceeding your limit, as even 50 calories may make a difference during this phase. If no mistake has been made, check with your physician to once again be sure that there is no hormonal deficiency. More elaborate diagnostic tests can be ordered if there is an indication of metabolic deficiency, but these disorders are quite rare, and if you simply give the 400 calorie intake a few more days, it is likely that you will show ketonuria again.

2. *Phase Two*

Once you are able to continue spilling intermittent ketones on 600 calories a day for a total of 4 weeks in Phase One, you enter Phase Two, where exercise is added along with an increase in your total calorie intake. The only exercise allowed at the start is walking, which uses 150 calories per hour at a rate of 2 mph, and 330 calories per hour at a rate of 4 mph. Start with 20 minute walks, and remember that they should be as uninterrupted as possible, since the aerobic benefit on your heart requires that you keep your pulse rate at a continuous elevated level. While the maximum heart rate is generally calculated at 220 beats per minute (bpm) minus your age, your target heart rate should range from 50-85% of this level, and for patients who are on VLCDs, compounded by the fact that obesity is already a strain on your heart, I suggest that you do not let your heart rate increase above 120 bmp. You can walk with a friend, listen to music on a recorder, or simply enjoy the pleasure of working your heart and skeletal muscle system. Do not try and immediately return to your pre-diet exercise routine, however, until you have adjusted to the ketosis which you are encountering as part of your weight-loss process. When you are tolerating the walks well, and not suffering from excessive appetite stimulation, you may begin to utilize other types of exercise, but I suggest you begin with walking since it is the easiest way to tune your muscles and assess your level of tolerance.

Although physical exercise is an important adjunct to any total health fitness agenda, I want to caution you about exercising too early in your *KetoFast* diet program, since it is one reason why many patients fail to lose weight in an otherwise proper calorie-restricted setting. While there is no question that a complete, well-rounded dietary health program must include the routine use of physical exercise for at least thirty minutes three times a week, it is not true that exercise must begin at the start of the agenda, before you have learned to control your appetite, and begun to lose weight. In fact, the opposite is true. Exercise is very invigorating, and it stimulates appetite, which is the normal reaction when you partially deplete the muscles of their mobile stores of glycogen and protein. This desire to replenish your energy preserves may make it impossible to follow the necessary calorie restriction at the early phase of calorie control. Although some physicians claim that exercise does not stimulate appetite, anyone who exercises on a regular basis knows that their feeling of vigor and strength is accompanied by a desire to eat. It is therefore important that you modify your calorie intake to a low enough level to assure weight loss before you begin to add exercise as a means to increase your catabolism of extra fat stores. I generally advise patients to complete Stage I, and at least 2 weeks of Stage II, before they embark on an exercise schedule.

To assess how much added exercise you will need to perform in order to increase your calorie intake above the levels suggested in Stage II and III, estimate your calorie usage by tables which are readily available on the internet. As a rule, walking will burn approximately 5.2 cal/min, bicycle riding

8.2 cal/min, swimming 11.2 cal/min and running 19.4 cal/min. The actual calories you consume will depend upon your weight (heavier people burn more calories), and your intensity (speed). A 30-minute leisurely walk will therefore utilize about 150 calories, while walking at a very brisk pace will burn about 190 calories. This same calorie expenditure will take place by walking up and down stairs for 15 minutes, bicycling 4 miles in 15 minutes, swimming laps for 20 minutes, or social dancing for 30 minutes. Do not expect your weight to melt away by exercise, however, for one pound of fat yields about 3500 calories of energy, so you would have to expend that amount of energy above your caloric intake to reduce your adipose tissue by one pound. This would take walking for 35 miles, bicycling for 60 miles at moderate speed, or doing low impact aerobics for almost eight hours, while eating nothing more than your standard intake for the day. You do not lose weight by exercise, you lose weight by eating fewer calories each day than you burn in your expenditure of energy. Once you have begun to effectively control weight loss, however, "continued exercise is associated with long-term maintenance of weight loss," as concluded by an expert panel of the American College of Sports Medicine.[154]

Once you have incorporated physical exercise into your daily routine, you can then begin to increase your caloric intake by 100-calorie increments every 1-2 weeks. Your goal is to eventually try and reach 1000 calories per day, while still maintaining a weight loss of 1-2 pounds per week. The more you exercise, the more quickly you can reach the goal of 1000 calories, but remember my cautionary statement earlier that this is not a race, and the goal is to achieve long-standing weight control, and not a rapid drain of fat that will ultimately reaccumulate. If you give your physiology time to adjust to stable fat catabolism, you will be less likely to regain the weight you have lost.

As food groups are added at this level, remember to try and increase the fiber content, so that proper digestion, as well as cancer prevention, is maintained. Much has been written about the importance of the fiber content of food in the last decade, and while the evidence is not incontrovertible, most physicians believe that a high fiber diet is associated with lower levels of cancer of the colon and rectum. Many of these food groups are also low in calorie content, so that they will fit in well with your calorie restriction, while still providing bulk to control your appetite.

In order to be sure your pilot light of fat catabolism is still lit, check yourself every two weeks by dropping your intake down to 500 calories for one day and be sure you are spilling some ketones in the urine. As long as you can verify that ketones are being produced, you can be assured that your system is burning fat. At some point in Phase Two, the amount of ketones being produced will decrease, so that the number of urines showing a positive reading will similarly decrease. This is due to two changes: the amount of fat in your body decreases, and therefore fewer fat cells will be burned, and the rate of fat burn will lessen, since the number of calories ingested increases. Although the urine no longer shows any evidence of ketones with the methodology being used, there is still some burning of fat that is undetectable metabolically. For most patients, this will not happen until you have reached a body weight that is about 40% above ideal weight. If your optimum weight is 170 pounds, this means that you should show ketones on a daily basis until you reach a weight of around 238 pounds. Although no ketones are appearing in your urine on a daily basis, you are still losing weight at an adequate level if you are maintaining a 1000 calorie diet. This will likely show up on the scale every two to three days, but if your weight loss stops altogether, return to the 500 calorie intake level for a few days and make sure ketones show up again, an indication that your are adequately burning fat. If there is significant ketonuria, you may have increased your calorie intake too quickly, and so slowly return to the prior level, but only increase by 100 calories every few days to keep the pilot light burning. Make sure you are not above 1000 calories per day, even if it is only a 50 calorie difference.

The duration of Phase Two, with calorie restrictions of below 1000 calories, has uniformly been shown to be safe for up to two months, although some researchers have suggested that it should be limited to one month.[155] A commentary in the Journal of the American Medical Association in 1990 claimed that 12-16 weeks was the "appropriate duration for the majority of patients."[156] This does not mean that you cannot remain at very restricted levels for longer than this period of time, but if you are going to continue severe restrictions beyond two months, it is best that you see your physician and reassess your metabolic state. Drs. Genuth, Castro, & Vertes from the Saltzman Institute for Clinical Investigation at Mt. Sinai Hospital of Cleveland used a 300 calorie diet for as long as 50 weeks in patients, and found that "no severe chemical derangements occurred."[157]

Before moving on to Stage III, let us stop for a moment and reflect on what has been accomplished in Stage II. You already have learned that the reason you are overweight is some undefined metabolic defect in your ability to mobilize fat. Where other people begin to catabolize fat at short intervals of time when they eat less than a specified amount, especially at night during sleep, your metabolic system may take up to 3-4 days to catabolize fat, even after a total water-fast. Because we cannot measure the extent of this deficiency by some blood test at this particular period of time, we have to follow your bodies response by measuring the amount of ketones being excreted into the urine as a reflection of how much fat is being catabolized. You started this process going by a zero-calorie water-fast which initiated fat burning after a delay which you have now recorded, and in Stage II you have modified the rate of this process by beginning to add back calories to a level that keeps weight loss proceeding at a slower, but still significant, rate. Your calorie intake has now reached a level of 1000 calories a day, and you are continuing to evaluate your ability to burn fat, both by the amount of weight you are losing, and also by rechecking the presence of ketones in your urine when you lower your calorie intake back down to 500 calories for a brief period of time. After a 2 month period of time, you are ready to utilize the lessons you have learned about estimating the calorie content of prepared dishes, and continue your weight loss program in the real world of food prepared by others.

C. Stage III

At this point in the dietary program, you have lost a significant amount of weight and must now embark on a maintenance program that will assure that your hormonal or enzymatic pathway deficiency will not cause you to regain significant amounts of weight over the next few months and years. This is a very critical part of *KetoFast*, for the primary problem with all diets is that without some type of modification of your lifestyle, you will regain 55-67% of the weight you lost within one year.[158] Where some obese patients are overweight because of easily modified lifestyle problems, your disorder is a genetic inability to readily burn fat as an energy source, making it more difficult for you to maintain a lower weight. You must therefore be constantly careful to assure that your "pilot light" of fat catabolism is always lit, so you can quickly return to your desired weight if you begin to regain excess pounds. Since we do not know the exact reasons for your physiologic abnormality, it is impossible to determine how quickly this undesired weight gain is likely to occur, and therefore the length of Stage III is indeterminate, and may last for many years. It is even possible that your metabolic system will never change, and that you will have to follow the precepts enclosed herein for the rest of your life, or until pharmacologic research comes up with a medication that solves your problem.

The primary goal of Stage III is to help you reach the calorie intake which is generally recommended for long-term use by the majority of diet programs, while continuing to assure that you can periodically burn fat cells by going on a 1-day water-fast. Your goal should be to reach 1200 calories per day for women, and 1500 calories per day for men. While such levels may support continued weight loss in most people, it is possible you will begin to gain weight at these levels, especially if you are not accurately measuring the portions of your food intake. If you find that you begin to regain weight when you reach this level, be sure to periodically reduce your intake and measure your urine ketone output, in order to reignite your consumption of fat stores. Do not get discouraged if this re-accumulation of weight happens, and remember that minor changes in your calorie intake can make major differences in your weight loss. Also realize that 50 fewer calories per day will result in a loss of 10 pounds over a year in normal individuals, and in you it may be even greater if it allows you to keep your pilot light for burning fat lit.

In addition to modifying your dietary intake for the first year, you should go on a 1- or 2-day water-fast each month, and check your urine for ketones. If you can show at least a trace of ketone after 24-48 hours, rather than 48-72 hours, you know that your system is no longer as resistant as it was when you were at your initial weight. Undertaking this water-fast each month should not be a difficult undertaking, since many people go on such a program once each week as a means of detoxifying their bodies, and providing spiritual sustenance. Self-control is a valuable tool to have for many stresses in your life, and honing your strength during a 1-day water-fast will help you handle many problems which heretofore led to an increased consumption of food.

If you do not show any ketonuria during this 1-day water-fast, don't panic, at least not yet. As long as your weight is not climbing, you are not significantly enlarging your fat cells, so all you have to do is stoke your fires of fat catabolism, and once again begin to reduce your stores of adipose tissue. For most people, this will involve increasing your amount of aerobic exercise so that you can burn up any stores of glycogen which may have developed during your increased caloric intake. Multiple studies have shown that persons treated by diet plus exercise are much more likely to maintain their weight loss than those who diet alone.[159] Although this is easier said than done, you can make exercise a priority in your weekly schedule if you only accept and believe in the system. Here are some hints to maintain success.

First of all, pick an exercise that can be done at home. This typically involves either a treadmill or stationary bicycle, but can include other apparatuses such as a rowing machine, skiing machine, or doing aerobic exercises to video tapes. While walking, running, or riding a bicycle outside will work in areas of the country subject to appropriate weather conditions, and working out at a health club or other indoor facility will provide a certain number of you with adequate times to work out, the majority of people will need to exercise at home if they are to continue a proper exercise program for a long period of time. You also will save travel time to and from a gym or other location. Also check out whether your place of work can provide a location for exercise, either before, during, or after the work day. Larger companies are competing with each other to build these types of facilities, and most provide access to entry level personnel, as well as the officers. Finally, take pride in what others are going to think about your new physique and energy level. Exercise will help you tone up and look good, and you will be able to notice a strength and endurance which will be obvious in a short period of time. Your overweight condition put your health at risk for a long period of time, but you also built muscles while you were carrying that weight around, and once you defat your system, you will be amazed at how strong you are compared to all those friends and neighbors who have been skinny all their life.

Secondly, as you begin to add more calories to your diet, it is important that you time your exercise to follow your meals, rather than precede. This is because studies have shown that you will obtain 30-50% more energy expenditure for up to three hours by a process known as "exercise-induced postprandial thermogenesis."[160] It is believed that this is due to the fact that eating stimulates the sympathetic nervous system, which stimulates the metabolic rate, and helps to burn fat. This benefit is especially advantageous in the late afternoon and evening, when your metabolism begins to wind down. For that reason, I believe it is better that you exercise late in the day, rather than in the morning when you first arise, during the early stages of Stage III. Once your weight is controlled, and your dietary intake is stable, you can adjust your exercise schedule to fit your own preferences.

VIII. CONCLUSION

I began this book with a bold statement: "This book may save your life, or the life of a loved one." I hope the pages which followed have outlined the reasons for my confidence. Not only do I contend that you are going to lose significant amounts of weight with the *KetoFast* program, I believe you are going to truly feel better, both physiologically and psychologically, by the advantages of fasting which has been proven to lower blood pressure and serum levels of glucose and cholesterol, while at the same time allowing you to sleep better, be more confident, and, if some of the alternative medicine claims are true, cleanse your body of noxious chemicals.

I want to stress, however, that first and foremost, this book is about losing weight, and not undergoing a life-changing philosophy. You have a metabolic deficiency which has caused you to retain excessive amounts of triglycerides in your fat cells, and you have proven to yourself that the reason is due to a delayed excretion of ketones in your urine during periods of calorie deprivation. You now know why you have been so frustrated over the years in attempting to control your weight. While this book does not provide a ready cure to your problem, it at least answers questions which have plagued you, and provides a methodology to assist in controlling the level of your weight by more than measurements on a scale each morning before breakfast. Until medical science isolates, and then produces, either the hormone or enzymatic deficiency which is responsible for your obesity, it is necessary for you to keep your catabolic utilization of adipose tissue at a level that can control your body weight. Obesity is not only dangerous to your health, it will get progressively worse unless you can control the relentless cycle of increased appetite and weight gain.

In order to continually ignite your pilot light of fat catabolism, you have to periodically undergo a water-fast so that your glycogen stores scan be depleted, allowing your body to shift to utilizing fat stores as an energy source. Once you are accustomed to this methodology, it is likely you will find benefits beyond that of weight loss alone, but for now your goal is to become comfortable with the technique, and then decide what other benefits may follow. Claims have been made that fasting can "improve or even cure various diseases: cardiovascular and circulatory diseases, diseases of digestive system, diseases of locomotor system including rheumatism, respiratory system diseases including asthma, and the early stage of malignant diseases like cancer."[161] The list has even been extended to include migraines and glaucoma, bulimia, diseases of the liver and biliary tract, Crohn's disease, ulcerative colitis, psoriasis, chronic eczema, fibroid tumors, nasal polyps, lipomas, and lagging libido.[162] The literature in this field is too expansive for me to outline in this book, and I am not going to suggest that anyone undergo the *KetoFast* diet simply to improve the status of their health, unrelated to their overweight status. I would point out, however, that short term water-fasts have been utilized by many health practitioners as an adjunct to the maintenance of good health, and that using VLCD supplementation is a well-researched, safe way to lose weight.

IX. 100-CALORIE RECIPES

I want to emphasize that I do not include recipes here simply to take up space and make the book larger so that the publisher can charge more money. It is very clear that one of the major problems in long-term weight loss programs is the likelihood that you will regain weight once the initial phase of your particular diet is over. It is generally not difficult to lose weight with almost every diet that has been published. Think of it: why would there be so many diet books published if there were not many people who succeeded with the precepts put forth? Losing weight is easy, keeping it off is difficult. This is why you must learn what it means to eat a smaller calorie portion of food when you start eating a more normal diet.

These recipes are intended to teach you how you can truly eat good-tasting food that is low in calorie, and still keep your total calorie intake below 1000 calories in Stage II, and 1200-1500 calories for the rest of your life. You will not learn enough by reading alone, and to be able to keep your weight off, you must take a hands-on approach. Do not worry if you have never cooked before, the recipes contained herein are simple, and the instructions are easy to follow. I have tried to include multiple taste sensations, and a wide variety of food types, so that you can choose the ones which fit your particular preference. Although there are many low-calorie products which are commercially available in the frozen food or canned section of the grocery store, I want you to learn how to eat properly, so that you can continue the process when you are outside of your home. When I rotated through Cook County Hospital in Chicago, Illinois, the medical interns had a simple standing rule about learning new techniques: see one, do one, teach one. This book is step one – you see what to do. Now you must move on to step two – do what it takes to cook a low calorie meal. I will leave step three up to you.

Once you are adept at preparing these recipes, feel free to take your calorie-counter, and devise your own menus. Be sure to pay attention to each additive, however, including oils, type of rice, pasta, or broth. Although I have repeatedly said that it is calories, and not the type of food you eat, which matters in the battle to lose weight, there is a new concept which categorizes carbohydrate-containing foods in the manner in which sugar is absorbed during the digestive process, and you may want to utilize this evaluation when choosing your particular recipe ingredients. This is known as the dietary glycemic index (GI), which is a system for classifying carbohydrate-containing foods according to how fast the body turns the food into glucose, thereby initiating an insulin response. For many years it was believed that the blood glucose response to the ingestion of carbohydrates was dependent upon the chain-length of the substance, giving rise to the suggestion that complex carbohydrates were healthier to eat than simple sugars like glucose. Dr. David J. Jenkins and his colleagues at the University of Toronto challenged this idea in 1981, however, and suggested instead that carbohydrates which break down rapidly during digestion raise the blood sugar more quickly that those that break down slowly, causing the insulin level in the blood to rise to higher levels, thereby increasing deposition of fat. The difference is due to the fact that there are two kinds of starches, amylose and amylopectin. They both have glucose rings linked together in long chains, but amylopectin chains also branch out on the sides, providing more surface area for the digestive enzymes to work on. High-GI meals, as defined by the two hour blood glucose response curve following the ingestion of a fixed portion of carbohydrate, will produce greater postprandial insulin concentrations than low-GI meals, and thereby may lead to greater accumulation of fat. High-glycemic foods are rated at 70 and up, moderate-glycemic foods are from 40-69, and low-glycemic foods are 39 and below. You can find a complete list of the GI index of foods at the database maintained by the University of Sydney in Australia at www.glycemicindex.com. The value of determining the glycemic index in choosing carbohydrate exchanges was endorsed by the Food and Agriculture Organization (FAO) of the United Nations and the World Health Organization (WHO) in 1997, and nutritionists throughout the world have begun to modify their recommendations accordingly.[163]

Foods which are in the low-GI range include most fruits and vegetables (but not root vegetables), legumes, oats, buckwheat, whole barley, All-bran, pumperknickel and rye bread, yoghurt, brown Basmati rice, noodles, and milk. High-GI foods include corn flakes, dates, jelly beans, soda, baked potato, white Jasmine rice (except for Uncle Ben's Converted Rice), table sugar, French bread, bagels, most popular cereals, Cream of Wheat, watermelon, doughnuts, French fries, parsnips, pretzels and white bread. Adding vinegar to the food will lower the GI, as will the presence of soluble dietary fiber, which can inhibit carbohydrate absorption. Recent studies suggest that consumption of an alcoholic drink prior to a meal reduces the GI of the meal by approximately 15%, but alcohol adds a caloric intake on its own, so I do not recommend you abide by this statistic. In addition, the ingestion of fats, acidic citrus fruits, and less refined breads will slow the absorption process, leading to a lowering of the glycemic index. This is why a slice of stoneground wholewheat bread has a GI of 53, while standard wholewheat bread is 67.

While many adherents have flocked to this theory, there is little controlled experimental data to prove the underlying thesis, and there is also a disturbing variation in published GI values for the same foods. This has been explained on differences which occur because of foods having different ingredients, being processed with a different method, and being ingested with other foods which may affect absorption. It is therefore important to look on the label of the foods you eat to see how much total carbohydrate is included, for that will raise the blood sugar significantly, even if the glycemic index is low. This is especially evident with soy milk, which generally has a low glycemic index, but may have significant amounts of carbohydrate, depending upon the manufacturer. It is nevertheless prudent, however, to consider utilizing these particular carbohydrates when developing your 100-calorie diet portions.

A further modification of this concept has been developed with the concept of the "glycemic load" (GL), which takes into account not only the rate at which the sugar in a food is absorbed, i.e. the glycemic index, but also how much sugar is actually contained within a food. This makes choosing a food more realistic, since you care more about how much sugar you are actually eating, and not only the rate of absorption. In general, a GL of 20 or more is high, 11-19 is medium, and 10 or under is low. Carrots, which have a high GI of 131, have a low GL of 10. This means you can safely eat carrots, despite their high GI rating. Air-popped popcorn also has a relatively high GI of 79, but an incredibly low GL of 4. Bean sprouts and grapefruit have both a low GI and low GL score, so are excellent additions to your diet. I suggest you research this concept in greater detail on your own, and try to choose foods with low GL content as much as possible.

One final bit of information which may prove helpful to those of you who are not experience in reading recipes, do not get hung up on the directions for spices. Everyone's palate is different, and the spice amounts which are included will not satisfy all tastes. Increase or decrease as desired, but for convenience, the following conversions may be helpful: 1 teaspoon = 5 milliliters; 1 tablespoon = 15 milliliters, or 3 teaspoons, or ½ ounce; 1 cup = 235 milliliters, or 8 fluid ounces, or 16 tablespoons; 1 pint = 473 ml, or 32 tablespoons, or 16 ounces.

BREAKFAST PORTIONS

1 LARGE BOILED EGG, 77 calories (1 serving)

Place egg in a medium saucepan and add enough cold water to cover the egg by about 1 inch. Bring to a boil, and then reduce the heat to low, so water temperature is just below simmering. Cover and cook for 2-3 minutes for soft-boiled egg, and 10-15 minutes for hard-boiled egg. Remove egg with a spoon and allow to cool slowly, or run under cold water.

1 SCRAMBLED EGG WITH SKIM MILK, 101 calories (1 serving)

vegetable cooking spray
1 egg, or 4 egg whites, lightly beaten
2 tablespoons skim milk
1 teaspoon chopped parsley
1 teaspoon minced chives
pinch of salt
pinch of freshly ground black pepper

Spray small nonstick skillet with vegetable cooking spray. Preheat skillet at medium heat and add ingredients. Cook for 3-4 minutes, stirring frequently.

HERB-SCRAMBLED EGG WHITES, 87 calories (1 serving)

vegetable cooking spray
3 egg whites, lightly beaten
1 cup arugula or baby spinach
1 garlic clove, minced
½ tomato, diced (may substitute scallions, leeks, spinach or mushrooms)
2 tablespoons chopped fresh basil
pinch salt
pinch freshly ground black pepper

Spray small nonstick skillet with vegetable cooking spray. Add garlic, and cook for 2 minutes over medium heat. Pour in the egg whites, tomato, basil, salt, and pepper, and cook for 4-5 minutes, stirring frequently.

SCRAMBLED EGG WHITES WITH TOFU, 80 calories (2 servings)

vegetable cooking spray
½ cup egg substitute, or 2 egg whites, lightly beaten
5 ounces water-packed firm light tofu, drained
1 ½ cups chopped spinach
1/8 teaspoon salt
1/8 teaspoon freshly ground black pepper

84

Spray a large skillet with vegetable cooking spray. Crumble the tofu and cook over medium-high heat, stirring continuously for 3 minutes. Add the spinach and cook for 1 minute. Whisk the eggs and add them to the skillet with the salt and pepper. Scramble together for 3 minutes.

RED AND YELLOW PEPPER EGG WHITE OMELETTE, 90 calories (2 servings)

vegetable cooking spray
1 teaspoon extra-virgin olive oil
6 egg whites, lightly beaten
1 sweet red pepper, thinly sliced
1 yellow pepper, thinly sliced
2 teaspoons grated Parmesan cheese
½ teaspoon dried basil
1/4 teaspoon freshly ground black pepper

Warm the olive oil in a medium nonstick frying pan over medium heat. Add the red and yellow peppers and cook, stirring frequently, for 5 minutes. Keep warm over low heat. In a small bowl, lightly whisk together the egg whites, basil, and black pepper. Coat a small nonstick frying pan with vegetable cooking spray and warm over medium-high heat for 1 minute. Add half of the egg mixture, swirl to evenly coat the bottom of the pan, and cook for 30 seconds. Carefully loosen and flip and cook for 1 minute. Sprinkle half the peppers over the eggs and fold to enclose the filling. Transfer to a plate and sprinkle with 1 teaspoon of the cheese. Repeat with the remaining mixture.

EGG WHITE FRITTATA, 89 calories (1 serving)

vegetable cooking spray
3 egg whites, lightly beaten
½ tomato, diced
1 tablespoon chopped fresh cilantro
1 tablespoon capers, rinsed
pinch salt
pinch of freshly ground black pepper

Spray a small nonstick frying pan with vegetable cooking spray and heat over a medium heat. Mix the egg whites, salt, and pepper in a small bowl and pour in the pan. Add the rest of the ingredients. Cook over medium heat for 2 minutes, turn and cook for 2 more minutes.

SCRAMBLED TOFU, 112 calories (2 servings)

½ tablespoon extra-virgin olive oil
3/4 cup mashed silken firm tofu (6 ounces)
½ cup sliced mushrooms

1/4 cup finely chopped green bell pepper
1 medium scallion, finely chopped
½ teaspoon minced garlic
1 plum tomato, cut into ½-inch cubes (about ½ cup)
1 tablespoon low-sodium soy sauce
½ tablespoon minced fresh flat-leaf parsley
½ tablespoon minced fresh basil, or 1/4 teaspoon dried basil
½ tablespoon minced fresh oregano, or 1/4 teaspoon dried oregano
1/4 teaspoon freshly ground black pepper

Heat the olive oil in a medium nonstick skillet over medium heat.
Add the mushrooms, bell pepper, scallions, and garlic. Cook, stirring
occasionally, until the vegetables are tender, about 4 minutes. Stir in the other
ingredients and cook for 3 minutes.

WAFFLES, 102 calories (4 servings)

1 cup unbleached all-purpose flour
1 1/4 teaspoons baking powder
1 cup nonfat milk
3 egg whites
2 ½ tablespoons unsweetened applesauce
½ teaspoon vanilla extract
pinch of salt

In a medium bowl, stir together flour, baking powder, and salt. In
another bowl, combine milk, 3 egg whites, applesauce, and vanilla, and whisk
to blend. Add the bowl ingredients together and stir to blend. Bake waffles on
a preheated waffle iron, either nonstick or lightly sprayed with vegetable
cooking spray.

CEREALS

A bowl of cereal in the morning, with skim milk, can provide a
satisfactory and healthy meal for under 100 calories, if you are careful to
choose from products which are free of added sugar ingredients. Cereals are a
good choice for breakfast in Stage II, as they provide beneficial fiber. The
following products are acceptable. Remember, however, that one cup of skim
milk has 90 calories, so use as little as possible.

Puffed Wheat (Quaker)	51 calories per cup
Puffed Rice (Quaker)	56 calories per cup
7 Whole Grain Puffs (Kashi)	70 calories per cup
Corn Flakes (Kellog)	79 calories per cup
Total (General Mills)	81 calories per cup
Shredded Wheat (Nabisco)	87 calories per cup
Wheaties (General Mills)	88 calories per cup

Corn Flakes (General Mills)	89 calories per cup
Cheerios (General Mills)	91 calories per cup
3/4 cup hot cooked oatmeal or oat bran	90 calories

For variance in taste, add 6-8 grapes, raspberries, blueberries, or blackberries, which contain about 4-5 calories per unit.

To customize your own breakfast with other choices during Stage II, pick from the following portions:

1 banana (6-inch)	80 calories
½ cup unsweetened blueberries	40 calories
1/4 cantaloupe (5-inch)	30 calories
½ medium grapefruit	40 calories
1 nectarine	67 calories
1 orange	62 calories
1 peach	42 calories
½ cup fresh pineapple chunks	40 calories
1 cup raspberries	60 calories
1 cup unsweetened strawberries	60 calories
1 tangerine	37 calories
½ whole wheat bagel, toasted	90 calories
1 slice mixed grain, white or whole wheat bread	65 calories
1 slice raisin bread, toasted	65 calories
1 slice pumpernickel or rye bread	80 calories
½ cup nonfat plain yogurt	45 calories

SAVORY SHAKES

As you build your calories during Stage II, you may find the need at times to have a quick ingestion of calories without a time commitment to make a salad or soup. These shakes will provide an excellent option throughout the day.

BANANA STRAWBERRY SHAKE WITH TOFU, 69 calories (2 servings)

½ cup soft tofu
½ lemon, juice of
½ banana
1 cup fresh strawberries
3 ice cubes or ½ cup crushed ice

Place ingredients in a blender and blend until smooth.

CARROT, APPLE AND GINGER SHAKE, 104 calories (1 serving)

2/3 cup carrot juice
½ cup apple wedges
1 tablespoon grated fresh ginger
1 teaspoon lemon juice
3 ice cubes or ½ cup crushed ice

In a blender, combine all of the ingredients and puree until thick and smooth.

ORANGE SUNSHINE SMOOTHIE, 89 calories (1 serving)

½ cup orange juice
1/4 cup plain non-fat yogurt
1 tablespoon Splenda
3 ice cubes or ½ cup crushed ice

In a blender, combine all of the ingredients and puree until thick and smooth.

PEACH SOY SMOOTHIE, 96 calorie (4 servings)

½ of a 16-ounce package frozen unsweetened peach slices (about 2 cups)
1 medium banana
1 cup vanilla soy milk or plain soy milk
1/4 cup frozen orange-pineapple juice concentrate, thawed
1 cup ice cubes

Place ingredients except for ice in a blender and blend until smooth. Gradually add the ice cubes and continue blending.

RASPBERRY BANANA COOLER, 66 calories (2 servings)

1 cup frozen raspberries (not in sugar syrup)
½ medium banana
1 cup lemon-lime soda
1 packet Equal
3 ice cubes or ½ cup crushed ice

Place ingredients in a blender and blend until smooth.

STRAWBERRY SMOOTHIE, 82 calories (4 servings)

2 ½ cup non-fat plain or vanilla yogurt
1/4 cup skim milk
4 packets Equal
2 cups frozen unsweetened whole strawberries
1 cup ice cubes

Blend the yogurt, milk, and Equal, and add berries, a few at a time, and continue to process until smooth. Add ice cubes, two at a time, and blend until slushy.

YOGURT-CUCUMBER SHAKE, 69 calories (1 serving)

½ cup fat-free yogurt
½ cup peeled, seeded, and sliced cucumber
3 tablespoons minced fresh dill
3 tablespoons minced red onion
1/4 teaspoon salt
2 ice cubes

In a blender, combine all of the ingredients and puree until thick and smooth.

To devise your own diet shake, be sure to use skim milk, which is only 85 calories for one cup (8 ounces), and provides excellent protein and low fat calories, along with calcium supplementation. A cup of whole milk, on the other hand, is 150 calories, lo-fat 2% is 120 calories, and lo-fat 1% is 102 calories. To make a 100-calorie portion with skim milk you can add 1/3-1/2 cup of your favorite fruit, and a dash of preferred extracts, such as vanilla, chocolate, and pineapple. Egg whites are another good source of protein, and add only 17 calories per egg.

SALADS

Salads are great 100-calorie choices, for they are low density in calories, and high in fiber content. In order to provide protein, and reach a 100-calorie portion on the lo-cal salad recipes, you can add 6 boiled shrimp (35 calories), ½ slice beef bologna (40 calories), 1 slice chicken bologna (44 calories), 1 slice turkey bologna (60 calories), 1 slice chicken breast (30 calories), 1 slice ham (22 calories), 1 slice pork olive loaf (60 calories), 1 slice roast beef (Hansel 'n Gretel, 30 calories), 1 slice salami (50 calories), 1 slice turkey breast (25 calories), ½ ounce almonds, cashews or filberts (10 nuts, 70 calories), 6 black or green olives (25 calories), 1 slice (1 ounce) reduced-calorie American cheese (50 calories), ½ cup 1% fat cottage cheese (82 calories), 1 slice Kraft free singles (45 calories), 1 slice part skim mozzarella cheese (72 calories), or 1 slice Weight Watchers cheese (50 calories). For added fiber, add 1 cup grated raw carrots (47 calories).

A number of these recipes call for the vegetables to be steamed. If you are uncomfortable utilizing the methods recommended, you can place the vegetables in a microwaveable dish with 3 tablespoons of water and cover tightly with microwave-safe plastic wrap. Microwave for about 3-4 minutes on high heat.

BASIC GREEN SALAD, 71 calories (4 servings)

4 cups torn green leaf lettuce
1 cup sprouts
1 cup tomato wedges
1 cup peeled, sliced cucumber
1 cup shredded carrots
½ cup chopped radishes
½ cup prepared lo-fat, sugar-free dressing of your choice

Toss the lettuce, sprouts, tomato, cucumber, carrots, and radishes in a large bowl with the dressing until the vegetables are coated. If desired, substitute lemon juice for the dressing, as the juice of one lemon has only 12 calories, while two tablespoons of lo-fat, sugar-free salad dressing usually contain about 70 calories.

ARUGULA AND RADICCHIO SALAD, 94 calories (4 servings)

2 bunches arugula (about 3 cups), stems discarded, thoroughly washed and cut into bite-size pieces
1 small head radicchio (about 5 ounces), halved, cored, leaves separated and washed, and cut into bite-size pieces
1 cup thinly sliced celery, strings removed
3 tablespoons minced Italian leaf parsley
1/4 cup red onion, minced
2 ½ tablespoons extra-virgin olive oil

½ teaspoon sugar
½ teaspoon coarse Kosher salt
½ teaspoon freshly ground black pepper
1 tablespoon balsamic vinegar

In a small bowl, add the parsley, onion, sugar, salt, pepper, and vinegar and stir to combine. Add oil, a little at a time, whisking until well-blended. In a salad bowl combine arugula, radicchio, and celery. Drizzle the dressing over and toss until well combined.

ASPARAGUS SALAD WITH CAESAR VINAIGRETTE, 70 calories (4 servings)

1 1/4 pounds asparagus spears (about 20 spears)
4 cups gourmet salad greens
1 garlic clove, minced
3 tablespoons tarragon vinegar
1 ½ teaspoons olive oil
1 teaspoon water
½ teaspoon anchovy paste
1/8 teaspoon freshly ground black pepper
1/4 cup garlic-favored croutons

Snap off tough ends of asparagus and remove scales. Steam for 4 minutes over boiling water, rinse under cold water and drain well. Stir the next 6 ingredients in a small bowl with a whisk. Arrange 1 cup greens on each of 4 plates, and top each with 5 asparagus spears. Drizzle the dressing over each serving and top with the croutons. Sprinkle with parsley if desired.

SOUTHWESTERN BLACK BEAN SALAD, 90 calories (3 servings)

1 cup canned or cooked black beans, drained
1/4 cup diced red onion
1/4 cup diced tomatoes
1/4 cup diced green bell pepper
1/4 cup chopped green onion
1/4 cup cooked corn kernels
½ tablespoon chopped fresh cilantro
2 tablespoons fine herb vinegar or seasoned rice vinegar
½ teaspoon chile powder
1/8 teaspoon sea salt
1/8 teaspoon freshly ground black pepper

Combine the beans, vegetables, and cilantro in a mixing bowl and toss gently. In a small cup, mix the vinegar, chile powder, salt, and pepper. Pour the dressing over the salad and mix well. Refrigerate for at least 30 minutes before serving.

MARINATED BROCCOLI AND CARROTS, 106 calories (4 servings)

1 large broccoli stalk, peeled and cut into spears
2 medium carrots, peeled and cut into 2 ½ x 1/4-inch sticks
1 large garlic clove, minced or pressed
1 teaspoon grated fresh ginger root
2 tablespoons canola or other vegetable oil
2 tablespoons rice vinegar
2 teaspoons soy sauce

In a large saucepan, cook the broccoli spears in boiling water for 2 minutes. Stir in the carrots and continue to simmer for 4 minutes. Drain and transfer to a serving bowl. Whisk the last 5 ingredients together in a small bowl and pour on the vegetables. Toss well and refrigerate, or set aside at room temperature, for 20 minutes before serving.

AFRICAN-SPICED BROCCOLI AND CAULIFLOWER SALAD, 57 calories (2 servings)

3/4 cup small broccoli florets
3/4 cup small cauliflower florets
½ cup diagonally sliced carrots
1/4 teaspoon ground ginger
1/4 teaspoon ground cumin
1/4 teaspoon ground coriander
1/8 teaspoon ground nutmeg
3 tablespoons fat-free cream
2 teaspoons cider vinegar
½ teaspoon honey
2 tablespoons sliced green onions
1/8 teaspoon salt
1/8 teaspoon dried crushed red pepper

Arrange the vegetables in a steamer basket over boiling water and cover and steam for 2 minutes. Rinse under cold water and drain well. Combine the vegetables with ginger, cumin, coriander, nutmeg, salt, and pepper in a small skillet and cook over medium heat for 2 minutes, stirring constantly. Combine with the other ingredients in a bowl and stir well.

WARM BROCCOLI AND RED ONION SALAD, 57 calories (4 servings)

4 cups broccoli florets
3 cups water
½ cup nonfat plain yogurt
2 tablespoons red wine vinegar
½ cup raisins
½ medium red onion, thinly sliced

Bring water to a boil in the bottom of a steamer. Steam broccoli over water for 3 minutes. Whisk the yogurt and vinegar together in a small bowl. Pour over the broccoli and toss with raisins and onion slices.

BRUSSELS SPROUTS, ORANGE, AND FENNEL SALAD, 102 calories (2 servings)

2 cups trimmed Brussels sprouts (about ½ pound)
3/4 cup thinly sliced fennel
2 small oranges, peeled, quartered and thinly sliced
2 tablespoons white wine vinegar
1 teaspoon grated orange rind
2 teaspoons water
1 teaspoon vegetable oil
1/4 teaspoon ground ginger
1/8 teaspoon salt
1/8 teaspoon freshly ground black pepper

Steam the Brussels sprouts in a steamer basket over boiling water for 8 minutes. Rinse with cold water and drain well. Place the Brussels sprouts, fennel, and oranges in a medium bowl. Mix the rest of the ingredients in a small bowl and then add to the salad and toss well.

CAESAR SALAD, 93 calories (4 servings)

4 cups (about 1 large bunch) romaine lettuce, cleaned and torn into pieces
2 tablespoons grated Parmesan cheese
2 tablespoons water
2 tablespoons red wine vinegar
1 teaspoon Worcestershire sauce
1 teaspoon lemon juice
1 tablespoon extra-virgin olive oil
1 clove garlic
1/4 teaspoon dry mustard
2 anchovy fillets, rinsed, and patted dry
1 cup croutons

Combine ingredients except lettuce and croutons in a food processor and blend until smooth. Pour over lettuce and toss well. Serve with 1/4 cup croutons over each portion.

SHREDDED CARROT SALAD, 60 calories (2 servings)

2 medium carrots, shredded (1 ½ cups)
1 small zucchini, shredded (1 cup)
1 medium bell pepper, chopped (1 cup)
1/4 cup fat-free Italian dressing

1/4 teaspoon freshly ground black pepper

Mix all ingredients in a bowl and serve chilled.

CAULIFLOWER AND BLACK OLIVE SALAD, 87 calories (4 servings)

4 cups (about 1 large) cauliflower, trimmed and broken into small flowerets
1 large Spanish onion, peeled and sliced into rings
2/3 cup black olives, stones removed and chopped
4 tablespoons extra-virgin olive oil
2/3 cups water
2 tablespoons lemon juice (½ lemon)
3 ½ tablespoons tomato paste
1/4 teaspoon salt
1/4 teaspoon freshly ground black pepper
2 tablespoons fresh chopped parsley

Heat the olive oil in a large saute pan and gently cook the cauliflower for 2 minutes. Remove the cauliflower and cook the onion in the same pan for 2 minutes. Return the cauliflower to the pan and add the lemon juice and water. Bring to a boil, reduce heat and simmer for 3 minutes. Remove the cauliflower and add the tomato paste and boil rapidly for one minute. Reduce heat and stir in the olives. Arrange the cauliflower on plates and spoon the olive sauce over the top. Serve chilled, sprinkled with the parsley.

THAI COLESLAW, 95 calories (4 servings)

6 cups shredded napa (about 1 small head, 1 pound) shredded Chinese cabbage
2 cups shredded red cabbage
1 cup shredded carrots
1 cup red bell pepper strips
2 tablespoon chopped dry-roasted peanuts
1 tablespoon chopped fresh cilantro
1 tablespoon chopped fresh mint
3 tablespoons fresh lime juice
3 tablespoons rice vinegar
2 tablespoons fish sauce
1 tablespoon water
1 tablespoon creamy peanut butter
1 teaspoon chile paste with garlic
1 garlic clove, minced

Combine the last seven ingredients in a large bowl and blend with a whisk. Add the other ingredients and toss gently to coat. Cover and marinate in refrigerator for 1 hour before serving.

VEGETABLE COLESLAW, 90 calories (4 servings)

2 ½ cups finely shredded green cabbage
1 1/4 cups finely shredded zucchini (1 medium)
1 ½ cups finely shredded jicama
1 finely shredded small carrot
1 cup fresh corn kernels, cooked
2 tablespoons chopped green onions
2 tablespoons toasted, shelled sunflower seeds
1 tablespoon chopped fresh cilantro
2 tablespoons extra-virgin olive oil
2 tablespoons lime juice
2 tablespoons white wine vinegar
1 teaspoon grated lime peel
½ teaspoon sugar
1/4 teaspoon chili powder
1/4 teaspoon salt
1/4 teaspoon freshly ground black pepper

Combine the first 7 ingredients in a large bowl and toss gently. Mix the other ingredients in a small bowl and then add to the slaw and mix well. Cover and refrigerate for 1 hour before serving.

MARINATED COLESLAW, 64 calories (4 servings)

2 cups coarsely shredded red or green cabbage
2 cups coarsely shredded white cabbage
1 cup thinly sliced cucumber (about 1 medium)
1 cup coarsely shredded carrot
½ cup diced purple onion
½ cup green pepper, cored and chopped
½ cup cider vinegar
1 tablespoon sugar
1 tablespoon Dijon mustard
1 tablespoon vegetable oil
2 teaspoons prepared horseradish
1/4 teaspoon salt
1/4 teaspoon freshly ground black pepper
1 teaspoon caraway seeds

Combine the first 6 ingredients in a large bowl and toss gently. Combine the other ingredients in a jar, cover tightly, and shake vigorously. Pour over the slaw and toss gently. Cover and chill for 8 hours before serving.

TOFU COLESLAW, 84 calories (4 servings)

4 cups thinly sliced green cabbage

1 cup grated carrot
3/4 cup finely diced celery
1 cup bean sprouts
1 cup reduced-fat firm tofu, drained (about 6 ounces)
1/4 cup low-fat mayonnaise
4 teaspoons rice vinegar
2 teaspoons prepared mustard
1 teaspoon sugar
2 garlic cloves
1/4 cup chopped fresh parsley
½ teaspoon salt
1/8 teaspoon freshly ground red pepper

Combine the first 4 ingredients in a large bowl. Combine tofu and next 7 ingredients in a blender and process until smooth. Add parsley and pour over the slaw mixture. Toss to coat, cover and chill for 1 hour before serving.

CRUNCHY ORIENTAL COLESLAW, 58 calories (4 servings)

1 ½ cups shredded red cabbage
1 ½ cups shredded napa cabbage
4 ounces snow peas, julienned
1 sweet red pepper, thinly sliced
½ cup thinly sliced radishes
½ cup low-sodium vegetable stock
3 tablespoons lemon juice
1 tablespoon low-sodium teriyaki sauce
3/4 teaspoon sesame oil
1 teaspoon cornstarch
1 tablespoon grated fresh ginger
2 teaspoons sesame seeds
1/4 teaspoon red-pepper flakes

In a large bowl, combine the first 5 ingredients. In a small saucepan, mix the next 5 ingredients and bring to a boil over medium heat, stirring frequently, and cook until slightly thick. Remove from heat and stir in the next 3 ingredients. Pour over the slaw and toss well. Cover and refrigerate for at least 1 hour before serving.

COUSCOUS SALAD, 108 calories (4 servings)

2 cups cooked couscous
2 cups diced fresh tomato
½ cup chopped fresh mint
½ cup minced red onion
½ cup diced cucumber
½ cup chopped fresh parsley

4 tablespoons lemon juice
1 large garlic clove, minced
½ teaspoon ground cumin
½ teaspoon ground coriander
½ teaspoon salt
1/4 teaspoon freshly ground black pepper

Prepare the couscous according to package directions. In a large bowl, combine all of the ingredients and toss gently to coat.

CRABMEAT SALAD, 107 calories (4 servings)

2 cans crabmeat (4 ounces each)
3 ounces daikon radish, peeled and chopped
½ large yellow bell pepper, chopped
2 scallions, chopped
1/4 cup black olives, chopped
1/4 teaspoon garlic powder
1/4 teaspoon ground coriander
½ teaspoon celery seed
2 tablespoons reduced-calorie mayonnaise
2 teaspoons Dijon mustard
1 tablespoon rice vinegar
1 medium tomato cut into 4 slices, ½-inch thick
½ teaspoon salt
1/4 teaspoon freshly ground black pepper

Drain crabmeat and place in a colander and rinse. Combine the other ingredients except for the tomato slices in a large bowl and mix well. Add the crabmeat and mix well. Chill for one hour before serving. Place upon tomato slices. If preferred, place upon celery stalks instead of tomatoes, but you will only save 4 calories.

CUCUMBER SALAD, 45 calories (3 servings)

2 large cucumbers, sliced diagonally crosswise
1 small onion, chopped
½ cup sliced radishes
1 clove garlic, minced
4 teaspoons rice wine vinegar
1 teaspoon reduced-sodium soy sauce
1 teaspoon sesame oil
1 packet Equal
1/4 teaspoon Kosher salt
1/8 teaspoon freshly ground black pepper

Whisk the last 7 ingredients in a large bowl. Add cucumbers, radishes, and onion and mix well. Allow to stand for 15 minutes and mix again before serving.

MARLENE'S CUCUMBER SALAD, 40 calories (2 servings)

2 large cucumber, thinly sliced
1 tablespoon extra-virgin olive oil
1 tablespoon rice vinegar
½ teaspoon sea salt
½ teaspoon onion powder
½ teaspoon garlic powder

Whisk the oil, vinegar, salt, onion powder and garlic powder in a medium bowl. Add the cucumbers and mix well. Allow to stand for 30 minutes before serving.

EGG WHITE SALAD, 96 calories (2 servings)

8 eggs
2 tablespoons minced onion
½ tomato, finely chopped
1 tablespoon low-fat mayonnaise
2 tablespoons Dijon mustard
1 teaspoon minced chives
1/4 teaspoon salt
1/8 teaspoon freshly ground black pepper
2 large lettuce leaves

Boil the eggs in salted water for 10 minutes. Immediately run the boiled eggs under cool water, crack, and peel away the egg shells while running under cold water. Separate the whites from the yolks and discard the yolks. Chop the egg whites in a large mixing bowl and then add the other ingredients except for the lettuce and mix well. Serve over lettuce, or celery if desired.

GAZPACHO SALAD, 51 calories (4 servings)

3 cups, seeded, chopped tomato
1 cup peeled, chopped cucumber
1 cup chopped green pepper
1/4 cup thinly sliced green onion
1/4 cup chopped purple onion
2 tablespoons minced fresh basil or 2 teaspoons dried basil
2 cloves garlic, minced
2 ½ tablespoons red wine vinegar
1 teaspoon extra-virgin olive oil
1 teaspoon Dijon mustard

1/8 teaspoon salt
1/8 teaspoon freshly ground black pepper

   Combine first 5 ingredients in a large bowl and toss gently. Combine
remaining ingredients in a small bowl and whisk until blended. Pour the
vinaigrette mixture over the vegetables and toss gently. Cover and chill for 1
hour before serving.

GREEN BELL PEPPER AND TOMATO SALAD, 91 calories (3 servings)

2 medium green bell peppers, cut in strips
1 medium tomato, diced
2 tablespoons extra-virgin olive oil
1 teaspoon lemon juice
1 clove garlic, minced
½ teaspoon paprika
1/4 teaspoon salt
3 cups shredded lettuce

   Place the peppers in a microwave-safe bowl and cover. Cook on high
for 5 minutes. Allow to cool and then combine with the remaining ingredients
except the lettuce. Mix thoroughly and cover and refrigerate for 1 hour.
Arrange 1 cup of lettuce on each of 3 salad plates and divide the mixture evenly
on top of the lettuce.

LEMON GREEK SALAD, 105 calories (4 servings)

1 medium unpared cucumber, thinly sliced
2 cups bite-size pieces spinach
2 cups bite-size pieces Boston lettuce
5 radishes, chopped
1/4 cup crumbled feta cheese
2 tablespoons sliced green onions (with tops)
10 pitted ripe black olives, sliced
1 medium tomato, cut into thin wedges.
2 tablespoons lemon juice
1 tablespoon dark olive oil
1 teaspoon sugar
1 teaspoon Djon-style mustard
1/8 teaspoon freshly ground black pepper

   Shake the lemon juice, olive oil, sugar, mustard and pepper in a
tightly covered container. Combine the cucumber, spinach, lettuce, radishes,
feta cheese, onions, olives, and tomatoes in a large bowl and add dressing. Toss
gently to coat.

GREEN BEAN AND CHERRY TOMATO SALAD, 51 calories (4 servings)

3/4 pound green beans, trimmed
3/4 pound cherry tomatoes, quartered
½ teaspoon chopped fresh oregano
1 ½ tablespoons red wine vinegar
½ tablespoon minced shallots
1 teaspoon extra-virgin olive oil
1/4 teaspoon salt
1/8 teaspoon freshly ground black pepper

      Cook beans in boiling water for 7 minutes. Drain and place beans, tomatoes, and oregano in a large bowl, and toss gently. Combine vinegar and shallots, stirring with a whisk, and let stand for 10 minutes. Add oil, salt, and pepper to the vinegar mixture, and stir with a whisk until well blended. Pour vinaigrette over bean mixture and toss well.

ISRAELI SALAD, 70 calories, (4 servings)

2 medium cucumbers, peeled and diced
2 medium tomatoes, cubed
1 small red onion, chopped
1 yellow pepper, diced
1 yellow summer squash, cubed
1/4 cup nonfat chicken broth
2 tablespoons extra-virgin olive oil
2 tablespoons lemon juice
1 large clove garlic, minced
1 tablespoon minced fresh basil or 1 teaspoon dried basil
½ teaspoon dried oregano
1/8 teaspoon salt
1/8 teaspoon freshly ground black pepper

      In a large bowl, combine the first 5 ingredients and toss gently. In a small cup, mix the rest of the ingredients and pour over the vegetables, tossing gently. Cover and marinate at room temperature for at least 1 hour before serving.

MESCLUN SALAD WITH CUCUMBER AND FETA CHEESE, 88 calories (2 servings)

6 cups mesclun (gourmet salad greens)
1 cup thinly sliced peeled English cucumber
2 tablespoons crumbled feta cheese
2 tablespoons thinly sliced green onions
2 tablespoons tomato juice
1 tablespoon rice vinegar

1 teaspoon extra-virgin olive oil
½ teaspoon sugar
1/4 teaspoon salt
1/8 teaspoon freshly ground black pepper

Whisk tomato juice, vinegar, olive oil, sugar, salt, and pepper in a small bowl. Combine mesclun, cucumber, feta cheese, and onions in a large bowl and add dressing, tossing gently to coat.

SHIITAKE AND ENOKI MUSHROOM CITRUS SALAD, 102 calories (4 servings)

1 ½ cups sliced shiitake mushroom caps (about one 3 ½-ounce package)
1 ½ cups orange sections
1 ½ cups thinly sliced cucumber
½ cup sliced radishes
1 package (3-ounce) enoki mushrooms
4 cups sliced romaine lettuce
1/4 cup vinegar
3 tablespoons orange juice
2 tablespoons light teriyaki sauce
1 tablespoon dark sesame oil
2 teaspoons peeled, minced fresh gingerroot
1 garlic clove, minced

Combine last 6 ingredients in a large bowl and stir well. Add first 4 ingredients and stir well and let stand for 5 minutes. Arrange 1 cup lettuce on each of 4 salad plates and spoon 1 cup of the orange mixture over each serving, and then divide the enoki mushrooms evenly among the salads.

MUSHROOM AND BLUE CHEESE SALAD, 112 calories (4 servings)

8 ounces mushrooms, thinly slice
1 ½ cups julienned snow peas
4 cups arugula leaves
1 cup coarsely chopped red leaf lettuce
3 tablespoons white wine vinegar
1 ½ teaspoons peanut oil
2 teaspoons coarse-grain mustard
1 teaspoon Dijon mustard
1/8 teaspoon freshly ground black pepper
2 cups seasoned croutons
2 tablespoons crumbled blue cheese.

In a large bowl, toss together the mushrooms, snow peas, arugula, and lettuce. In a small bowl, whisk together the next 5 ingredients. Pour over the salad. Toss to mix well, and sprinkle with the croutons and blue cheese.

CRUNCHY PEA SALAD, 101 calories (4 servings)

2 cups shelled green peas
1 cup diced cucumbers
½ cup thinly sliced radishes
1/4 cup thinly sliced green onions
2 tablespoons rice vinegar
1 tablespoon extra-virgin olive oil
1 tablespoon honey
1/4 teaspoon salt
½ teaspoon coarsely ground black pepper

  Place peas in a steamer basket over boiling water, cover and steam for 6 minutes. Rinse under cold water and drain well. Add peas to the other vegetables in a large bowl. Combine vinegar and remaining 4 ingredients in a small bowl and stir with a whisk. Pour over vegetable mixture and toss well.

PINTO BEAN SALAD, 96 calories (4 servings)

1 15-ounce can pinto beans, rinsed and drained
½ cup thinly sliced red onion
1 teaspoon extra-virgin olive oil
1 tablespoon red wine vinegar
1 teaspoon minced fresh rosemary
1 garlic clove, minced
1/8 teaspoon salt
1/8 teaspoon freshly ground red pepper
4 large lettuce leaves

  Combine the ingredients except for the lettuce in a bowl and toss well. Serve over a large lettuce leaf.

RICE AND CORN SALAD, 100 calories per serving (4 servings)

1 cup cooked rice, preferably Basmati
½ cup cooked sweet corn kernels
2 ounces fat-free cheddar cheese, shredded
1 fresh tomato, finely diced
2 green onions, white and green parts, thinly sliced
½ small red bell pepper, finely diced
1/4 teaspoon ground cumin
1/4 cup fresh cilantro, chopped
1 tablespoons green chilies, chopped
3 tablespoons fat-free Italian dressing
Radicchio lettuce leaves, washed and chilled

In a large bowl, whisk the Italian dressing and cumin and then add all the other ingredients except for the lettuce. Stir and toss until it is well combined and then cover and refrigerate for at least one hour. Place one small mound of the mixture on a lettuce leaf and serve. May use other types of lettuce, although it is more visually appealing, and easier to eat, with Radicchio.

WILD RICE AND RADISH SALAD, 100 calories (2 servings)

1 cup cooked chilled wild rice
1/4 cup finely chopped yellow bell pepper
1/4 cup thinly sliced radishes
1 scallion, minced
½ tablespoon prepared horseradish
½ tablespoon Dijon mustard
2 tablespoons dry white wine

Combine the rice, yellow bell pepper, radishes, and scallion in a bowl and toss well. Mix the horseradish, mustard and wine in a small bowl, and pour over the salad. Toss to coat well.

ROMA SALAD WITH CAPERS, OLIVES, AND MOZZARELLA, 100 calories (3 servings)

4 cups sliced plum tomatoes (about 10 tomatoes)
2 cups thinly sliced red onion
1/4 cup coarsely chopped fresh basil
2 tablespoons capers
1 tablespoon chopped pitted kalamata olives
½ teaspoon coarse sea salt
1/4 teaspoon freshly ground black pepper
2 tablespoons balsamic vinegar
1 teaspoon extra-virgin olive oil
1/4 cup (1 ounce) shredded fresh mozzarella cheese

Combine the first 7 ingredients in a large bowl and toss gently. Combine the vinegar and oil in a small bowl, whisk, and then drizzle over the mixture. Toss gently and then sprinkle with the cheese.

SHRIMP SALAD, 102 calories (4 servings)

1 cup water
20 medium shrimp, peeled and deveined
1/4 teaspoon salt
1/4 teaspoon garlic powder
1/4 teaspoon ground oregano
1/4 teaspoon freshly ground black pepper

16 large lettuce leaves (romaine or leaf)
3 cups chopped iceberg lettuce
½ cup finely chopped celery
½ cup finely chopped green bell pepper
½ cup finely chopped red bell pepper
½ cup finely chopped dill pickle
½ cup finely chopped onions
2 large pimento-stuffed olives, chopped
4 medium tomatoes, quartered

In a large skillet, bring the water to a boil and add the shrimp, salt, garlic powder, oregano, and pepper. Reduce the heat to medium and simmer for 3 minutes. Remove from heat and drain the shrimp, but save the cooking liquid. In a bowl, toss together the chopped iceberg, celery, red and green bell pepper, pickle, onions, and olives. Divide equally and place on top of 4 overlapping lettuce leaves arranged on 4 salad plates. Top each with 5 shrimp and 2 tablespoons of the cooking liquid. Garnish with the tomatoes.

SPINACH, ARUGALA AND RADISH SALAD, 88 calories (4 servings)

4 cups spinach, arugula, and lettuce
3/4 cup thinly sliced red radishes
1/4 cup shredded mint leaves
1/4 cup pine nuts, toasted
3/4 tablespoon extra-virgin olive oil
½ tablespoon honey
2 tablespoons rice vinegar
1 ½ teaspoons Dijon mustard
½ teaspoon salt
1/4 teaspoon freshly ground black pepper

Combine the first 4 ingredients in a bowl and mix well. Whisk the other ingredients in a small bowl and add to the salad and toss lightly.

SPINACH WITH SPROUTS SALAD, 90 calories (5 servings)

8 ounces fresh spinach torn into bite-size pieces
1 can (16 ounces) bean sprouts, rinsed and drained, or 2 cups fresh sprouts
1 can (8 ½ ounces) water chestnuts, drained and sliced
1 cup croutons
2 tablespoons low-sodium soy sauce
2 tablespoons sesame seeds, roasted and crushed
2 tablespoons lemon juice
½ teaspoon honey
1 tablespoon finely chopped onion
1/4 teaspoon freshly ground red pepper

Combine the soy sauce, sesame seeds, lemon juice, honey, pepper and onion in a tightly covered container and shake well. Place the spinach, bean sprouts, and water chestnuts in a large bowl, and toss well. Add the dressing and toss gently to coat well. Sprinkle with croutons when serving.

MANGO SPINACH SALAD, 90 calories (4 servings)

6 cups torn spinach
3 cups torn Boston lettuce
1 cup cubed mangoes
1 tablespoon poppy seeds
2 tablespoons balsamic vinegar
2 tablespoon rice wine vinegar
1 tablespoon honey
1 ½ teaspoons coarse-grain mustard
pinch of ground cardamom
1/8 teaspoon freshly ground black pepper

In a large bowl, combine the spinach, lettuce, mangoes, and poppy seeds. In a small bowl, whisk the other ingredients and then pour over the salad and toss well.

SUGAR SNAP PEA SALAD, 61 calories (4 servings)

4 cups water
1 cup trimmed sugar snap peas
4 cups torn romaine lettuce pieces
3/4 cup julienned jicama
1/4 cup very thin wedges red onion
1/4 cup apple juice
1 teaspoon Dijon mustard
1 tablespoon honey

Bring water to boil in a saucepan. Drop in peas and immediately remove from heat. Plunge the peas into cold water and drain. Mix the mustard, honey, and apple juice in a cup. Combine the snap peas, lettuce, jicama, and onion in a bowl. Pour dressing over the salad and toss well.

TABBOULEH, 103 calories (4 servings)

½ cup bulgur
3/4 cup coarsely chopped cucumber
1/4 cup snipped parsley
4 green onions, sliced (½ cup)
3 tablespoons lemon juice
2 tablespoons water
1 tablespoon extra-virgin olive oil

1 teaspoon dried mint, crushed
1/8 teaspoon garlic salt
1/8 teaspoon freshly ground black pepper
1 large tomato, chopped

Rinse bulgur in a colander with cold water. Drain, and combine bulgur, cucumber, parsley, and onions in a medium mixing bowl. In a screw-top jar, combine lemon juice, water, olive oil, mint, garlic salt, and pepper. Cover jar and shake to mix well. Pour over the bulgur mixture and toss to coat. Cover and chill for at least 4 hours. Stir tomato into the mixture before serving.

TOFU SALAD, 88 calories (2 servings)

4 ounces firm tofu, drained and mashed
½ cup quartered cherry tomatoes
4 large romaine lettuce leaves
2 tablespoons light mayonnaise or tofu mayonnaise
2 teaspoons chopped fresh cilantro
1/4 teaspoon salt
1/8 teaspoon freshly ground black pepper

Combine the ingredients except for the lettuce in a small bowl and mix thoroughly. Place equal portions in the lettuce leaves and fold the sides. Wrap in plastic wrap and refrigerate for 1-2 hours before serving.

TOMATO, BASIL AND FRESH MOZZARELLA SALAD, 60 calories (4 servings)

6 (1/4-inch-thick) slices yellow tomato (1 ½ pounds)
6 (1/4-inch-thick) slices red tomato (1 ½ pounds)
1/4 cup (1 ounce) shredded fresh regular or low-fat mozzarella cheese
1/4 cup thinly sliced fresh basil
½ teaspoon freshly ground black pepper

Basil sauce
1 cup loosely packed fresh basil leaves
1/3 cup vegetable broth
1/4 cup balsamic vinegar
1 teaspoon sea salt

To prepare basil sauce, cook 1 cup basil leaves in boiling water for 15 seconds, drain, and plunge into ice water. Drain and pat dry. Combine basil and broth in a blender and process until smooth. Let stand at room temperature and strain through a fine sieve into a bowl. Add vinegar and salt, stirring with a whisk. Arrange the tomato slices alternately on a large platter, red and yellow, and drizzle with basil sauce. Sprinkle with cheese and pepper and top with sliced basil.

TOMATO, SWEET ONION, AND CORN SALAD, 89 calories (4 servings)

2 large tomatoes, thinly sliced
½ cup thinly sliced Vidalia or sweet onion
½ cup chopped cucumber
1 cup fresh white corn kernels (about 2 ears)
½ cup basil leaves
1 tablespoon chopped fresh basil
2 tablespoons white balsamic vinegar
2 teaspoons extra-virgin olive oil
1 ½ teaspoon Dijon mustard

   Toss the first five ingredients in a large bowl. Whisk the fresh basil, vinegar, olive oil, and mustard in a small bowl and drizzle over the salad. Toss gently and serve.

TOMATO AND ZUCCHINI SALAD, 65 calories (3 servings)

1 large tomato, coarsely chopped
1 small zucchini, thinly sliced
2 tablespoons sliced green onion
1 teaspoon snipped fresh basil or 1/4 teaspoon dried basil, crushed
2 tablespoons reduced-calorie Italian dressing
3 large Romaine lettuce leaves
2 tablespoons crumbled feta cheese or shredded part-skim mozzarella cheese

   In a medium mixing bowl, combine the first 5 ingredients and toss lightly to mix. Place a large lettuce leaf on each of 3 salad plates, and add the salad. Sprinkle each serving with some of the cheese

TUNA-VEGETABLE SALAD, 109 calories (4 servings)

½ cup chopped celery
½ cup chopped seeded cucumber
½ cup shredded carrot
2 tablespoons sliced green onion
1 6 ½-ounce can low-sodium chunk light or white tuna, drained and broken into chunks
4 medium tomatoes, sliced
½ cup fat-free mayonnaise dressing or salad dressing
1 ½ teaspoons snipped fresh dill or ½ teaspoon dried dillweed
½ teaspoon finely shredded lemon peel
1/8 teaspoon garlic powder
1/8 teaspoon freshly ground black pepper

   In a medium mixing bowl, combine the celery, cucumber, carrot, and green onion. Stir in the dressing, dill, lemon peel, garlic powder, and pepper.

Gently fold in tuna. Cover and chill for 1-4 hours. To serve, divide the sliced tomatoes among 4 plates and spoon the tuna mixture over the slices.

SPICY TURKEY AND CABBAGE SALAD, 100 calories (2 servings)

3/4 cup julienned, cooked turkey breast (about 3 ounces)
2 ½ cup shredded green cabbage
1 cup shredded red cabbage
½ cup julienned carrots (about 1 small)
1/4 teaspoon toasted sesame oil
1/4 teaspoon chile sauce
1/4 cup seasoned rice wine vinegar
2 tablespoons soy sauce

Combine the turkey, cabbages, and carrots in a large bowl. In a small bowl, whisk the sesame oil, chile sauce, vinegar, and soy sauce, and then drizzle over the salad and toss well. Refrigerate for 30 minutes before serving.

WATERCRESS AND SPROUT SALAD, 78 calories (2 servings)

4 cups trimmed watercress
1 cup bean sprouts
1 tablespoon sesame seeds, toasted
2 tablespoons low-sodium soy sauce
1 tablespoon rice vinegar
1 tablespoon water
1 tablespoon sesame oil

Combine last four ingredients in a medium bowl and stir well with a whisk. Add the watercress and sprouts and toss gently. Sprinkle the sesame seeds on the top of the salad.

WATERCRESS-BIBB SALAD WITH APPLES AND BLUE CHEESE, 61 calories (3 servings)

4 cups torn Bibb lettuce
1 ½ cups trimmed watercress
1 cup thinly sliced Granny Smith apples (about ½ pound)
1/8 cup (½ ounce) crumbled blue cheese
3 tablespoons apple juice
1 tablespoon cider vinegar
1 tablespoon finely chopped shallots
2 teaspoons Dijon mustard
1 teaspoon vegetable oil
1/4 teaspoon salt
1/4 teaspoon freshly ground black pepper

108

Combine the last 7 ingredients in a jar, cover tightly, and shake vigorously. Place in refrigerator for at least 2 hours. Combine the lettuce, watercress, apples, and blue cheese in a bowl and add dressing. Toss well.

With all of these salads, in order to provide more protein and omega-3 fatty acids, feel free to sprinkle any of the following seeds over the top of your portion: flaxseed (linseed), chia seeds, pumpkin seeds, sesame seeds, and sunflower seeds, and add about 25 calories per teaspoon. If you are constipated by the small portions of the meals you are eating, flaxseed is an especially good choice, since it tends to increase bowel movements when taken in larger amounts. The lignans in flaxseed have been postulated to benefit the heart and possess anti-cancer properties, in addition to lessening the severity of diabetes.

To add extra calories with high protein, you can use anchovies, which average 10 calories apiece.

COOKED VEGETABLE DISHES

GRILLED ASPARAGUS, 36 calories (4 servings)

vegetable cooking spray
1 1/4 pound asparagus spears (20 spears)
3 tablespoons balsamic vinegar
2 tablespoons fresh lemon juice
1 tablespoon extra-virgin olive oil
1 tablespoon low-sodium soy sauce
½ teaspoon freshly ground black pepper

   This dish is low enough in calories that you can add a slice of meat product as described below and have a good 100-calorie starter meal. Snap off touch ends of asparagus and combine all ingredients except cooking spray in a large zip-top plastic bag. Seal and marinate for 30 minutes. Remove asparagus and place on grill rack coated with cooking spray. Discard the marinade. Grill for 5 minutes on each side.

THAI ASPARAGUS, 63 calories (4 servings)

1 tablespoon peanut oil
1 1/4 pound asparagus spears, sliced on a diagonal, separating stalks and tips (20 spears)
4 large scallions, sliced thin
2 teaspoons grated peeled fresh ginger
2 tablespoons thinly sliced fresh lemon grass
1/4 teaspoon minced or ground dried red chile
4 tablespoons vegetable stock
1 tablespoon fresh lime juice
1 tablespoon soy sauce
1 tablespoon minced fresh mint
1/4 cup chopped fresh cilantro
1/4 teaspoon salt

   Set a wok over high heat. Add the oil and swirl to coat the inside of the pan. Add the scallions and stir-fry briefly. Add the ginger, lemongrass, and chile, stir and then add the asparagus gradually, stalks first. Add stock, 1 tablespoon at a time, and stir-fry until the asparagus is tender, about 5 minutes. Add the lime juice, soy sauce, mint, salt and cilantro and toss well.

LEMONY ASPARAGUS AND NEW POTATOES, 105 calories (4 servings)

3/4 pound fresh asparagus spears, cut into 2-inch lengths (12 spears)
8 whole tiny new potatoes, cut into quarters (about 10 ounces)
2 teaspoons extra-virgin olive oil
1/4 cup water

110

3/4 teaspoons snipped fresh thyme or 1/4 teaspoon dried thyme, crushed
½ teaspoon finely shredded lemon peel
½ teaspoon salt

      In a 2-quart covered saucepan, cook the quartered potatoes in a small amount of boiling water for 10 minutes. Add the asparagus, and cook, covered, for 8 minutes. Drain and transfer to a serving bowl. Combine the other ingredients in a small bowl and then add to the vegetables, tossing gently to coat.

ASPARAGUS WITH MUSTARD SAUCE, 37 calories (4 servings)

1 pound fresh asparagus spears, trimmed and cut into 1-inch pieces (16 spears)
1/4 cup water
½ tablespoon Dijon mustard
½ tablespoon lemon juice
1/8 teaspoon salt
3/4 teaspoon mustard seeds
½ teaspoon extra-virgin olive oil

      Put asparagus and water in a microwave-save bowl and cover. Microwave on high for 10 minutes, stirring every 3 minutes. Drain and set aside. In a small bowl, combine mustard, lemon juice, and salt. Toast the mustard seeds in olive oil in a large skillet for 1 minute, stirring frequently. Add asparagus and mustard mixture, and cook for 2 minutes.

ASPARAGUS AND PEAS, 75 calories (4 servings)

½ teaspoon sesame oil
6 ounces sugar snap peas, trimmed and cut diagonally
6 ounces snow peas, trimmed and cut diagonally
6 ounces asparagus spears, trimmed and cut diagonally (6 spears)
1 tablespoon sesame seeds
1 teaspoon low-sodium Worcestershire sauce
1 garlic clove, minced
1 tablespoon finely chopped fresh ginger
1/8 teaspoon salt
1/4 teaspoon red pepper flakes

      Briefly heat the sesame oil in a nonstick wok and then add the garlic, ginger, red pepper flakes, and salt. Stir-fry for 1 minute. Add the sugar snap peas, snow peas, and asparagus and stir-fry for 5 minutes. Stir in the Worcestershire sauce, and stir-fry for 1 minute. Sprinkle with sesame seeds and serve.

TURKEY-WRAPPED ASPARAGUS SPEARS, 105 calories (3 servings)

3/4 pound asparagus spears, trimmed (12 spears)
12 thin slices skinless deli turkey (about 5-ounces)
½ cup fat-free, or soy mayonnaise dressing
1 teaspoon chopped fresh tarragon, or 1/4 teaspoon dried, crumbled tarragon
1/8 teaspoon garlic powder
1/8 teaspoon grated lemon zest
dash of cayenne pepper

      Stir together the mayonnaise, tarragon, garlic powder, lemon zest, and cayenne in a small bowl, cover, and refrigerate for 3 hours. Fill a Dutch oven with about 4 inches of water and bring to a boil over high heat. Cook the asparagus for 3 minutes, remove and plunge immediately into a bowl of ice water. Drain well and pat dry. Spread 1 tablespoon of the tarragon sauce (aioli) on a slice of turkey and place the asparagus spear on top. Roll up jelly-roll style and repeat with the other slices.

KOREAN BEAN THREAD NOODLE STIR-FRY, 79 calories (4 servings)

2 teaspoons canola or vegetable oil
1 2-ounce package bean thread noodles, cut into 3-inch lengths
2 cups quartered fresh mushrooms
1 cup shredded cabbage
1 cup sliced carrots, cut into 2-inch slivers
½ cup scallions, cut in half lengthwise and cut into 3-inch lengths
1 teaspoon minced garlic
½ teaspoon chili powder
½ cup vegetable broth
1 tablespoon dark soy sauce
1 cup mung bean sprouts
1 teaspoon sesame oil
2 teaspoons white sesame seeds

      Place the noodles in a large bowl and pour boiling water over the noodles to cover. Let the noodles soak while you prepare the rest of the ingredients. In a large wok or skillet, heat the oil over medium-high heat and then stir-fry the garlic and chili powder for 10 seconds. Add the mushrooms, cabbage, carrots, and scallions and stir-fry for 2 minutes. Drain the noodles, and add them to the pan. Stir-fry for 30 seconds. Pour in the broth and soy sauce and stir-fry for 30 seconds. Remove from the heat and stir in the bean sprouts and sesame oil. Transfer to a serving platter and sprinkle with the sesame seeds.

ROASTED BEETS AND ONIONS, 103 calories (3 servings)

1 pound (about 1 bunch) beets with tops

2 small red onions (½ pound), not peeled
1 tablespoon extra-virgin olive oil
1/4 cup chicken broth
1/8 cup balsamic vinegar
½ teaspoon brown sugar
½ teaspoon fresh thyme
1/8 teaspoon salt
1/8 teaspoon coarsely ground black pepper
½ tablespoon chopped fresh parsley.

Preheat oven to 400^0. Trim all but 1 inch of stems from beets and place beets and onions in nonstick oven-safe skillet or baking pan. Drizzle with oil and roast, shaking occasionally, for 1½ hour. Transfer vegetables to a plate and when cool, peel beets and onions and place in a bowl. Combine broth, vinegar, sugar, and thyme in the same skillet. Heat to boiling, stirring and scraping bottom of skillet, for 5-7 minutes, or until reduced to about 1/8 cup. Stir in salt and pepper, cool, and pour over vegetables. Toss until coated and sprinkle with parsley.

PICKLED BEETS, 36 calories (4 servings)

vegetable cooking spray
One 16-ounce can sliced beets
½ small onion, sliced and separated into rings
2 tablespoons tarragon vinegar or cider vinegar
1/8 teaspoon freshly ground white pepper
3 packets Equal

Drain the beets and reserve ½ of the liquid. Spray a medium nonstick skillet with vegetable cooking spray and place over medium heat. Add the beets, reserved liquid, onion rings, vinegar, and white pepper. Cook for 3 minutes, stirring often. Remove from heat and stir in the Equal.

STIR-FRIED BOK CHOY, 52 calories (4 servings)

2 pounds (about 1 head) bok choy
1 shallot, sliced
1 tablespoon extra-virgin olive oil
1 garlic clove, crushed
1 tablespoon thinly sliced ginger
2 tablespoons soy sauce
½ teaspoon oyster sauce

Separate bok choy stalks from leaves, and cut both into ½-inch-thick slices. In 10-inch skillet, heat oil over medium-high heat. Add garlic, ginger, and shallot and cook for 1 minute. Add bok choy stalks and cook, stirring frequently, for 4 minutes. Add bok choy leaves, and stir-fry for 2 minutes. Stir in soy sauce and oyster sauce and remove from heat.

STEAMED BOK CHOY WITH GINGER DRESSING, 45 calories (2 servings)

1 pound bok choy, cut into 2-inch pieces
1 tablespoon white wine vinegar
2 teaspoons Dijon mustard
2 teaspoons soy sauce
1 teaspoon sugar
½ teaspoon extra-virgin olive oil
1 small clove garlic, finely chopped
1 tablespoon fresh ginger, finely chopped

Place bok choy in a steamer basket over boiling water. Steam for 10 minutes. Combine the other ingredients in a jar with a tight-fitting lid and shake vigorously. Transfer bok choy to a bowl and add dressing. Toss well and serve.

BROCCOLI AND CORN, 70 calories (3 servings)

1 package (10-ounce) frozen broccoli cuts or flowerets
1 cup frozen whole kernel corn
1 medium onion, chopped (½ cup)
½ cup water
2 teaspoons chopped fresh or ½ teaspoon dried basil leaves
½ teaspoon chicken bouillon granules
1 clove garlic, finely chopped
1 jar (2 ounces) diced pimentos, drained

Put all ingredients in a 1-quart saucepan and heat to boiling. Reduce heat to low, cover, and simmer for 5 minutes.

BRAISED BROCCOLI WITH GARLIC, 85 calories (3 servings)

1 pound broccoli raab
1 1/4 tablespoons extra-virgin olive oil
1 clove garlic, crushed, or 1 tablespoon from a jar
1/4 teaspoon Kosher salt
1/4 teaspoon freshly ground black pepper

Clean the broccoli, removing discolored leaves and bottom stems. Keep the florets. Peel the stems with a potato peeler and cut them into 3-inch lengths. Wash and drain thoroughly in colander. Steam the broccoli stems and florets over a steamer for 5 minutes, or in the microwave oven. In a medium saute pan, heat oil over medium-high heat. Lower to low heat and cook garlic until lightly golden. Remove from heat and add the broccoli and then cook

114

over medium-high heat for 5 minutes, or until stems are barely tender. Turn heat to high and cook another 2 minutes, or until stems are extremely tender. Season with salt and pepper and serve.

BROCCOLI WITH YOGURT, 40 calories (3 servings)

3 cups broccoli florets
1/4 cup nonfat plain yogurt
1 clove garlic, minced
2 teaspoons Dijon mustard
2 teaspoons lemon juice
1/8 teaspoon freshly ground black pepper

Steam the broccoli florets for 5 minutes. Whisk together the yogurt, mustard, lemon juice, garlic, and pepper in a small glass bowl, and then spoon over the broccoli and serve.

BROCCOLI AND PEPPERS, 64 calories (4 servings)

1 pound broccoli, cut into flowerets
1 red or yellow sweet pepper, cut into 1-inch pieces
2 tablespoons reduced-calorie margarine
1 teaspoon finely shredded lemon peel
1 tablespoon lemon juice
1/8 teaspoon freshly ground black pepper

Place broccoli and sweet pepper in a steamer basket over simmering water. Steam, covered, for 8 minutes. Arrange vegetables on a serving platter. In a small saucepan, melt the margarine. Stir in the next 3 ingredients and drizzle over the vegetables.

BROCCOLI STEMS AND PEAS, 90 calories (4 servings)

vegetable cooking spray
2 cups peeled broccoli stems
2 cups fresh green peas or 1 package (10 ounces) frozen
5 scallions, sliced
½ teaspoon dried marjoram
2 teaspoons fresh parsley, chopped
½ cup orange juice

Heat a nonstick skillet sprayed with vegetable cooking spray over medium heat. Add the broccoli and ½ of the orange juice, cover, and simmer for 5 minutes. Add the peas, scallions, marjoram, and remaining orange juice , stir and cook uncovered for 4 minutes. Sprinkle with parsley before serving.

BRUSSEL SPROUTS WITH GARLIC AND GINGER, 80 calories (4 servings)

1 pound Brussels sprouts, ends trimmed
1 ½ cups vegetable stock or water
1 tablespoon finely minced garlic
1 tablespoon grated fresh gingerroot
1 teaspoon grated lemon zest
1 ½ teaspoon anise seed
½ teaspoon salt
1/4 teaspoon freshly ground black pepper

Cut the Brussels sprouts in half, and then into very thin strips. This should make about 3 cups. Bring 1 cup of vegetable stock to a simmer in a large saute pan and add the sprouts, garlic, ginger, and lemon zest. Cook, uncovered, over high heat, stirring often for 6 minutes. Add more broth as needed. Stir in anise seed and season with salt and pepper.

BRUSSELS SPROUTS WITH PROSCIUTTO, 110 calories (4 servings)

1 pound Brussels sprouts, ends trimmed
1 tablespoon extra-virgin olive oil
2 ounces prosciutto, or lean cooked ham, chopped
1 teaspoon finely shredded lemon peel
1 tablespoon lemon juice
1/4 teaspoon kosher salt
1/8 teaspoon freshly ground black pepper

Cut the Brussels sprouts in half, and cook them in boiling lightly salted water in a covered large saucepan for 7 minutes. Drain well and place aside. Add oil to the same saucepan and head over medium-high heat. Add the sprouts and other ingredients, stir well, and cook for 1-2 minutes.

BRUSSELS SPROUTS AND MANDARIN ORANGES, 107 calories (3 servings)

2 cups trimmed fresh Brussels sprouts, halved, or 1 package (10 ounces) frozen, thawed
1 tablespoon unsalted butter
1 teaspoon crushed, toasted cumin seen
1 teaspoon mustard seed
1/4 teaspoon salt
1/4 teaspoon freshly ground black pepper
½ cup chopped onion
1 garlic clove, minced
2 large mandarin oranges, peeled and segmented, or 1 can (11 ounces) mandarin segments, drained

Pour ½ cup of water into a medium saucepan and bring to a boil. Add the brussels sprouts and cook 5 minutes. Drain and put aside. Melt the butter in a large nonstick skillet over high heat and stir in the next 4 ingredients. Add the brussels sprouts, onion, and garlic, and cook 3 minutes, stirring frequently. Add the orange segments, and cook 1 minute, stirring frequently.

BULGAR PILAF, 100 calories (4 servings)

1 teaspoon extra-virgin olive oil
1 small onion, chopped (1/4 cup)
1 medium carrot, cut into thin bite-size strips
½ cup bulgur wheat
1 ½ cups chicken broth
½ garlic clove, minced
1 teaspoon soy sauce
1 teaspoon Worcestershire sauce
½ teaspoon dried oregano
1/4 teaspoon freshly ground black pepper

In a small saucepan, heat olive oil and add onion and cook over medium heat for 3 minutes. Add bulgur and carrots and stir well. Add broth, garlic, oregano, soy sauce, Worcestershire sauce, and pepper and bring to boil. Cover, reduce heat to low, and simmer 14 minutes, or until all the liquid has been absorbed. Let stand for 5 minutes before serving.

CABBAGE, OLIVES AND CAPERS, 96 calories (4 servings)

6 cups (about 1 small head, 1 pound) trimmed, cored, thinly sliced savoy cabbage
2 teaspoons extra-virgin olive oil
1 packet Equal
1 cup chicken broth
1 tablespoon rinsed capers
8 kalamata olives, pitted and chopped
1/4 teaspoon salt
1/4 teaspoon freshly ground black pepper

Combine the cabbage, olive oil, and Equal in a large nonstick skillet. Cover and cook over low heat for 15 minutes, stirring occasionally. Increase the heat to medium and add the other ingredients. Cook, uncovered, for 15 minutes, stirring occasionally.

NAPA CABBAGE STIR-FRY, 106 calories (4 servings)

6 cups (about 1 small head, 1 pound) trimmed, cored, and thinly sliced napa (Chinese) cabbage
1 cup shredded carrots (about 2)

6 green onions, chopped
1 tablespoon light sesame oil
2-inch piece of fresh ginger, peeled and cut into 2 x 1/8 inch strips
4 garlic cloves, thinly sliced
1 tablespoon seasoned rice vinegar
½ teaspoon salt
1/4 teaspoon ground red pepper

In nonstick 12-inch skillet, heat oil over medium-high heat. Add ginger and garlic and cook, stirring frequently for 2 minutes. Add cabbage, carrots, salt, and pepper and stir-fry for 4 minutes. Add onions and vinegar and stir-fry 1 minute.

NAPA CABBAGE AND BAMBOO SHOOTS IN BLACK BEAN SAUCE, 90 calories (2 servings)

2 cups shredded napa or Chinese cabbage
1 can (8 ounces) bamboo shoots, drained
4 ounces firm tofu, drained and cut into bite-size cubes
2 tablespoons fermented black bean sauce
1 tablespoon water

Place the cabbage in a microwave-safe bowl. Combine the black bean sauce with 1 tablespoon of water in a small bowl and pour over the cabbage. Cover with a lid or vented plastic wrap and microwave on High for 3 minutes. Stir in the bamboo shoots and tofu and microwave on High for 2 minutes. Serve immediately.

SWEET AND SOUR CABBAGE, 70 calories (4 servings)

6 cups (about 1 small head, 1 pound) thinly sliced red cabbage
2 teaspoons extra-virgin olive oil
1 medium red onion, sliced thin
4 large garlic cloves, minced
2 tablespoons balsamic vinegar
1/4 teaspoon salt
1/8 teaspoon freshly ground black pepper

Set a wok over medium-high heat. Add the oil and tilt the pan to coat the inside. Add the onion and stir-fry for 2 minutes. Stir in the garlic, and gradually add the cabbage, continuing to stir-fry for several minutes until the cabbage is cooked but still slightly crisp. Remove from heat and add the other ingredients. Toss thoroughly and serve hot or cold.

CABBAGE WITH ZUCCHINI AND SESAME SEEDS, 75 calories (4 servings)

6 cups (about 1 small head, 1 pound) thinly sliced Savoy cabbage
1 tablespoon toasted sesame seeds
1 teaspoon extra-virgin olive oil
3 cups finely chopped zucchini
1/4 cup rice vinegar
1/4 cup low-sodium soy sauce
1 teaspoon chili paste with garlic
1/8 teaspoon freshly ground black pepper

Heat olive oil in a large nonstick skillet over medium-high heat, add zucchini and cook 3 minutes, stirring frequently. Add cabbage and next 4 ingredients, cover and reduce heat to medium, and cook 6 minutes. Stir in sesame seeds, and add 1 tablespoon of chopped fresh mint if desired.

ORANGE-GINGER CARROTS, 67 calories (4 servings)

1 16-ounce package peeled baby carrots
1 green onion, thinly sliced
2 tablespoons orange juice
1 tablespoon honey
3/4 teaspoon grated fresh ginger
½ teaspoon salt
1 tablespoon snipped fresh parsley

In a covered large saucepan, cook the carrots and onions in a small amount of boiling water for 4 minutes. Drain well. In a small bowl, stir together the orange juice, honey, ginger, and salt. Drizzle over carrots and toss to coat. Sprinkle with parsley, and, if desired, orange peel.

SESAME CARROTS AND GREEN BEANS, 100 calories (2 servings)

1 large carrot, halved lengthwise and sliced thin on a diagonal
½ pound green beans, sliced on a diagonal
2 medium scallions, sliced on a diagonal
6 tablespoons vegetable stock
1 tablespoon natural soy sauce
1 teaspoon dark sesame oil
1 tablespoon toasted sesame seeds

Add the stock to a wok and heat to boiling over high heat. Add the carrot and green beans, cover, and cook for 4 minutes, stirring occasionally. Stir in the scallions and remove the wok from the heat. Add the other ingredients and toss thoroughly.

COLD DIJON CARROTS, 86 calories (4 servings)

4 cups baby carrots
1 clove garlic, minced
1 tablespoon water
1 tablespoon extra-virgin olive oil
2 tablespoons Dijon mustard
1 tablespoon whole-grain mustard

Cook the carrots in boiling water for 5 minutes. Drain the carrots and run them under cold water, allowing them to cool for 10 minutes. In a small bowl, whisk the other ingredients together and pour them over the carrots, mixing completely.

INDIAN-STYLE CAULIFLOWER, 71 calories (4 servings)

1 head cauliflower, cut into florets (about 4 cups)
4 green onions, sliced into 1-inch pieces
1 small red or green pepper, cut into 1-inch pieces
1 tablespoon vegetable oil
1/4 cup chicken broth
½ teaspoon dry mustard
1/4 teaspoon ground turmeric
1/4 teaspoon ground cumin
1/8 teaspoon ground coriander
1/8 teaspoon freshly ground red pepper

In a bowl, combine the mustard, turmeric, cumin, coriander, and pepper and set aside. Heat olive oil in a wok or large skillet over medium-high heat. Add cauliflower and stir-fry for 3 minutes. Add green onions and sweet pepper and stir-fry for 1 ½ minutes. Reduce heat to medium and add mustard mixture. Cook and stir for 30 seconds and then carefully stir in broth. Cook and stir for 1 minute.

CAULIFLOWER SUPREME, 96 calories (4 servings)

vegetable cooking spray
1 head cauliflower, cut into florets (about 4 cups)
1/3 cup water
½ cup non-fat plain yogurt
½ cup reduced-fat sharp cheddar cheese
½ teaspoon dry mustard
Dash Cayenne pepper
½ teaspoon salt
1/4 teaspoon freshly ground black pepper

Cook cauliflower in water, covered, in microwave oven at high for 8 minutes. Drain and transfer to a baking dish coated with vegetable cooking spray. Combine yogurt with other ingredients and spread over the cauliflower. Bake, uncovered, for 9 minutes.

CAULIFLOWER AND BROCCOLI ROAST, 92 calories (4servings)

2 cups broccoli florets
2 cups cauliflower florets
5 cloves garlic, peeled and halved
2 tablespoons extra-virgin olive oil
½ teaspoon salt
1/4 teaspoon freshly ground black pepper
1 teaspoon grated Parmesan cheese

Preheat oven to 450^0. Toss broccoli, cauliflower and garlic with olive oil and spread on a baking sheet. Bake for 20 minutes, stirring once or twice. Season and sprinkle with Parmesan cheese before serving.

COLLARDS WITH YOGURT, 105 calories (3 servings)

1 pound fresh collard greens, trimmed, and chopped
½ cup diced onion
1/3 cup plain nonfat yogurt
1 tablespoon vegetable oil
1 tablespoon Dijon mustard
½ teaspoon salt

Place the greens in a large pot of boiling salted water and cook 10 minutes. Drain and set aside. Heat the oil in large nonstick skillet over medium heat. Add the onion, cover, and cook 3 minutes. Stir in the greens and salt. Reduce the heat and add the yogurt mixed with the mustard. Cook 5 minutes.

TOMATO-STUFFED EGGPLANT WITH FETA, 108 calories (4 servings)

1 medium eggplants, cut in half lengthwise (about 1 pounds)
3/4 cups (1/4-inch thick) sliced plum tomato (about 2 tomatoes)
½ tablespoon extra-virgin olive oil
½ tablespoon chopped fresh rosemary
½ tablespoon chopped fresh basil
1/8 teaspoon salt
1/8 teaspoon freshly ground black pepper
1 garlic clove, minced
3/4 cups crumbled feta cheese

Preheat oven to 500°. Place cut eggplant on a baking sheet and place tomato slices between eggplant slices. Brush oil over eggplant and sprinkle with rosemary and the next 4 ingredients. Bake for 15 minutes and then sprinkle with cheese and bake for another 4 minutes. Garnish with basil sprigs, if desired.

STEAMED JAPANESE EGGPLANT WITH SPICY GREEN SAUCE, 45 calories (4 servings)

12 ounces Japanese eggplant, cut into 3 x ½ inch sticks (about 5 cups)
½ cup minced green onion
3 tablespoons water
1 teaspoon extra-virgin olive oil
2 tablespoons low-sodium soy sauce
2 tablespoons rice vinegar
1 teaspoon grated peeled fresh ginger
1 teaspoon chile paste with garlic

Steam eggplant in a microwaveable dish with 3 tablespoons water covered, for 3 minutes. Combine other ingredients in a small bowel and stir well. Drizzle the eggplant with the sauce, and garnish with cilantro leaves, if desired.

CURRIED EGGPLANT, 108 calories (3 servings)

1 medium eggplant, peeled and cut into 1-inch cubes
4 plum tomatoes, diced
1/4 cup plain soy yogurt
1 teaspoon ground cumin
1 tablespoon curry powder
1/8 cup water
½ tablespoon vegetable oil
½ large onion, chopped
3 garlic cloves, minced
1 ½-inch piece fresh ginger, minced
1/8 teaspoon salt
½ teaspoon cayenne pepper

Steam eggplant cubes in a steamer basket over boiling water for 10 minutes and set aside. Over high heat, in a large saute pan, heat the oil and saute the onion for 7 minutes. Add the garlic and ginger, and cook for another 30 seconds. Mix the cumin, cayenne, salt, and curry powder in the water and add to the pan with the eggplant and tomatoes, and simmer for 5 minutes. Stir in the yogurt and simmer for 10 minutes. Serve warm or chilled.

122

EGGPLANT, OLIVES, AND PINE NUTS IN BELGIAN ENDIVE, 75 calories
(4 servings)

1 small eggplant (8 ounces)
1 ½ teaspoons extra-virgin olive oil
3 kalamata or Gaeta olives, chopped
2 teaspoons toasted pine nuts
1/4 teaspoon lemon juice
1/4 teaspoon salt
1/4 teaspoon freshly ground black pepper
12 Belgian endive leaves
1 teaspoon chopped parsley

Preheat the oven to 425^0. Pierce the eggplant in 4 places with a fork and place in a baking pan. Roast for 25 minutes, turning once or twice. Remove from oven and let cool. Cut the eggplant in half lengthwise and scrape out the pulp, discarding the stem and skin. Finely chop the eggplant and place in a medium mixing bowl. Gradually add the oil, stirring vigorously. Stir in the next 5 ingredients and then spoon the mixture onto the wide end of the endive leaves. Sprinkle with the parsley.

TASTY COOKING GREENS, 80 calories (1 serving)

vegetable cooking spray
1 cup chopped Swiss chard, woody stems trimmed
½ cup chopped kale, woody stems trimmed
2 cups chopped mustard greens, woody stems trimmed
3 teaspoons minced fresh garlic
1 teaspoon white wine vinegar
½ teaspoon freshly ground black pepper

Place the Swiss chard, kale, and mustard greens in boiling water for 5 minutes, and then immediately put into ice cold water, drain, and set aside. Spray an 8-inch nonstick skillet with vegetable cooking spray and heat over medium-high heat. Add the garlic and saute for 1 minute. Add the greens and sprinkle with the vinegar and pepper and stir for one minute.

GREEN BEANS WITH GARLIC VINAIGRETTE, 90 calories (3 servings)

1 pound (about 4 cups) green beans, trimmed
1/4 cup sliced almonds, toasted
½ tablespoon fresh thyme leaves

Vinaigrette
½ teaspoon grated lemon rind
1 tablespoon fresh lemon juice
2 teaspoons extra-virgin olive oil

2 garlic cloves, minced
1 teaspoon Dijon mustard
½ teaspoon salt
1/4 teaspoon freshly ground black pepper

Cook green beans in a large pot of boiling water for 4 minutes and drain well. Place in a large bowl. Prepare the vinaigrette in a small bowl and add to the beans and toss well to coat. Sprinkle with almonds and thyme.

GREEN BEANS WITH LEMON AND BROWNED GARLIC, 86 calories (3 servings)

1 pound (about 4 cups) green beans, trimmed
3/4 cup water
2 ½ teaspoons extra-virgin olive oil
3 garlic cloves, minced
3 tablespoons fresh lemon juice
1/8 teaspoon salt
1/8/ teaspoon freshly ground black pepper

Bring water to a boil in a nonstick skillet. Add green beans and cook 3 minutes. Drain and cool. Heat oil in skillet over medium heat, add beans and garlic and saute 1 minute. Add lemon juice, salt, and pepper and saute 1 minute.

GREEN BEANS PROVENCALE, 72 calories (4 servings)

1 pound (about 4 cups) green beans, cut into 2-inch pieces
1 ½ teaspoon extra-virgin olive oil
1cup thinly sliced sweet white onions
4 garlic cloves, crushed
2 cups plum tomatoes, seeded and thinly sliced (about 3/4 pound)
2 tablespoons chopped fresh basil or 2 teaspoons dried basil
1/8 teaspoon dried thyme
1/4 teaspoon salt
1/8 teaspoon freshly ground black pepper

Arrange green beans in a steamer basket over boiling water, cover and steam for 5 minutes. Drain. Heat olive oil in a large nonstick skillet over medium-high heat. Add onions and garlic and saute 1 minute. Add beans and saute 3 minutes. Add tomatoes and remaining ingredients and saute 2 minutes.

LEMON-GARLIC KALE, 41 calories (4 servings)

6 cups chopped kale, stems removed
1 medium onion, chopped,
2 cloves garlic, minced

124

2 tablespoons low-sodium chicken broth
3 tablespoons lemon juice
½ teaspoon ground black pepper

Heat the broth in a large skillet. Add the onion and garlic and saute for 2 minutes. Add kale and lemon juice, reduce heat to low, and cook for 8 minutes. Season with pepper and stir well.

TOMATO-GARLIC LENTILS, 61 calories (4 servings)

2 cups dried lentils
2 medium tomatoes, finely chopped
3 ½ cups water
2 tablespoons low-sodium tomato juice
1 tablespoon lemon juice
2 garlic cloves, minced

Heat tomato juice in a large saucepan. Add garlic and saute for 1 minute. Add tomatoes and saute for 5 minutes. Stir in the water and lentils. Bring to a boil, reduce heat, cover, and simmer for 30 minutes. Stir in lemon juice.

MUSHROOM MEDLEY, 105 calories (4 servings)

1 tablespoon extra-virgin olive oil
½ cup chopped onion
10 ounces sliced white mushrooms
8 ounces shitake mushrooms, stemmed and halved
6 ounces oyster mushrooms, trimmed and halved
1 teaspoon chopped fresh rosemary
1 tablespoon minced garlic
1/4 cup beef broth
½ teaspoon salt
1/4 teaspoon freshly ground black pepper

Heat the olive oil in a large nonstick skillet over medium-high heat. Add the onion and cook 1 minute. Add the mushrooms and rosemary and cook in a mound shape for 11 minutes, stirring occasionally. Add the garlic, salt, and pepper and cook for 3 minutes. Pour in the broth and cook for 2 minutes. If you cannot buy separate types of mushrooms, use 5 packages of mixed wild or domestic mushrooms, but be careful to maintain the same total weight.

GRILLED PORTOBELLO MUSHROOMS, 80 calories (4 servings)

vegetable cooking spray
4 large portobello mushrooms (about 2 pounds), washed with stems removed
1 tablespoon extra-virgin olive oil

125

3 tablespoons strained fresh lemon juice
½ teaspoon coarse Kosher salt
½ teaspoon freshly ground black pepper
3 tablespoons tender top green part of scallions
2 tablespoons minced parsley

Preheat charcoal grill sprayed with vegetable cooking spray, or broiler with tray 4 inches from the heat. Lightly brush mushroom caps with olive oil, and place on grill with cap sides down. Grill for 3 minutes, turning mushrooms once. Flip each mushroom and brush undersurface with olive oil. Transfer mushrooms to a cutting board and slice into ½-inch strips. Drizzle with lemon juice, and season with remaining ingredients.

PEAS IN TOMATO SHELLS, 80 calories (5 servings)

1 package (10 ounces) frozen green peas
5 medium tomatoes (about 1 ½ pounds)
2 tablespoons finely chopped green onions (with tops)
1 tablespoon snipped fresh dill week or 1 teaspoon dried dill weed
1/8 teaspoon freshly ground black pepper
2 tablespoons reduced-calorie sour cream

Remove stem ends from tomatoes and then remove the pulp from the wall of each tomato, leaving the bottom ½-inch thick. Cut a thin slice from the bottom of each tomato to prevent tipping, if necessary. Heat oven to 350^0. Separate peas under running cold water and drain well. Mix peas, onion, dill weed, and pepper. Place tomatoes in ungreased pie plate, 9 x 1 1/4 inches. Fill tomatoes with pea mixture and bake uncovered for 25 minutes. Top with sour cream if desired.

PEA POD STIR FRY, 63 calories (4 servings)

2 teaspoons vegetable oil
8 ounces green beans, trimmed
4 ounces snow pea pods, trimmed and strings removed
4 ounces sugar snap peas, trimmed and strings removed
½ cup thinly sliced carrot (1 medium)
1 garlic clove, finely chopped
1 tablespoon soy sauce
4 cups water
1 teaspoon salt

In a 12-inch skillet, combine 4 cups water and salt and heat to boiling over high heat. Add green beans and cook 3 minutes. Drain, wipe skillet dry, and heat oil over high heat. Add green beans and cook, stirring frequently, for 2-3 minutes, or until green beans begin to brown. Add snow pea pods, sugar peas, carrot, and garlic and stir fry for 1 minute. Stir in soy sauce and remove from heat.

PEPPERS STUFFED WITH POLENTA, 99 calories (4 servings)

2 6-ounce green or red bell peppers, cored, cut in half lengthwise, and seeded
½ cup yellow cornmeal
2 cups water
1/8 teaspoon salt
1/8 teaspoon freshly ground black pepper
1 teaspoon extra-virgin olive oil
4 teaspoons freshly grated Parmesan cheese

Preheat broiler. Put pepper halves, cut side down, on a baking sheet and place it under the broiler for 7 minutes, or until the skins start to turn black. Place peppers in a bowl and cover with a plastic wrap for 10 minutes. Remove peppers and peel off charred skin. In a 3-quart saucepan, bring the water and salt to a steady simmer. Turn heat to medium and add the cornmeal in a thin, constant stream. Stir continuously while adding cornmeal to prevent lumps from forming. Add the olive oil and cook for 20 minutes, stirring frequently. Preheat oven to 425° F. Place peppers, cut side up, on the baking sheet and fill each with the polenta. Sprinkle each with 1 teaspoon of the cheese. Bake for 7 minutes.

RATATOUILLE, 80 calories (3 servings)

1 teaspoon extra-virgin olive oil
½ cup diced yellow onion (about 1 medium)
½ cup diced zucchini (about 1 small)
½ cup diced yellow squash (about 1 small)
½ cup diced eggplant (about ½ small)
½ cup diced red bell pepper (about 1 small)
½ cup diced green bell pepper (about 1 small)
½ cup diced portobello mushroom, gills removed (about 1 medium)
1 ½ cup peeled, chopped fresh tomatoes, or 1 14-ounce can
1 tablespoon minced garlic
1 tablespoon balsamic vinegar
1 teaspoon dried thyme, dried oregano, or dried basil
½ teaspoon sea salt
1/4 teaspoon freshly ground black pepper

Heat a large saute pan over medium-high heat and add the olive oil to lightly coat the bottom of the pan. Saute the vegetables for about 5 minutes, or until they begin to soften, and then add the remaining ingredients and simmer for ten minutes. Feel free to modify the vegetables to your liking.

GARLIC-TOMATO RICE, 102 calories (4 servings)

1 teaspoon extra-virgin olive oil
1 cup long-grain rice, rinsed and drained
1 1/4 cup vegetable broth
2 garlic cloves, minced
1 small onion, finely diced
1 teaspoon tomato paste
1 tomato, seeded and diced
fresh parsley for garnish

In a large nonstick skillet, heat the oil over medium heat and add the garlic and onion and saute 7 minutes. Add the rice and stir until the grains are coated. Mix the broth with the tomato paste until blended and stir the mixture into the rice. Simmer for 8-10 minutes, or until the rice has absorbed the liquid. Stir the diced tomato gently into the rice and garnish with the parsley.

BASMATI RICE WITH PEAS, 100 calories (4 servings)

1 pound peas, shelled, or 10-ounce package frozen tiny peas
1 cup Basmati rice
2 cups and 2 tablespoons vegetable stock
½ small onion, finely chopped
1 garlic clove, minced
½ teaspoon dried basil
½ teaspoon fine sea salt
½ teaspoon freshly ground black pepper

Heat the 2 tablespoons vegetable stock in a 4-quart saucepan, and add the onion, garlic, and basil. Cook 2 minutes over low heat. Add the 2 cups of stock, rice, salt, and pepper and cover and cook over low heat for 20 minutes. Stir in the peas and cook 5 minutes more.

BROWN RICE PILAF, 60 calories (4 servings)

1 cup water
1 teaspoon instant chicken bouillon granules
1 cup sliced fresh mushrooms
3/4 cup quick-cooking brown rice
½ cup shredded carrot
3/4 teaspoon snipped fresh marjoram or 1/4 teaspoon dried marjoram, crushed
Dash freshly ground black pepper
1/4 cup thinly green onions
1 tablespoon snipped fresh parsley

In a medium saucepan, stir together the water and bouillon granules and bring to boiling. Stir in the next 5 ingredients and return to boiling.

Reduce heat, simmer, covered, for 12 minutes. Remove from heat and let stand for 5 minutes. Add the onions and parsley and toss lightly.

SPAGHETTI SQUASH WITH GARLIC AND PARMESAN, 100 calories (3 servings)

1 tablespoon extra-virgin olive oil
1 spaghetti squash
2 cloves garlic, minced
3 tablespoons grated Parmesan cheese
1/8 teaspoon salt
1/8 teaspoon freshly ground black pepper

Preheat oven to 350^0. Pierce the shell of the squash with a fork and bake, uncovered, for 45 minutes. Turn the squash over and bake for 30 minutes. Cut the squash in half and cut in half and remove the seeds. Remove the spaghetti strands with a fork and set aside. Saute the garlic in oil in a nonstick pan for 1 minute. Add the squash, salt and pepper and toss in the hot pan for 3 minutes. Sprinkle with Parmesan cheese before serving.

SPINACH SUPREME, 60 calories (serves 2)

vegetable cooking spray
2 cup fresh spinach leaves
1 cup chopped tomatoes
½ cup chopped onions
½ cup chopped green beans
2 teaspoon minced fresh garlic
1 teaspoon lemon juice
½ teaspoon freshly ground black pepper

Heat a nonstick skillet over medium heat and spray with vegetable cooking spray. Add the tomatoes and cook for 3 minutes, stirring occasionally. Add the onions, green beans, and garlic, and cook for 4 minutes. Add the spinach and cook for 30 seconds. Add the lemon juice and pepper, and stir well.

SPINACH WITH PINE NUTS, 95 calories (4 servings)

4 teaspoons extra-virgin olive oil
1 pound well-rinsed coarsely chopped spinach leaves
4 large garlic cloves, minced
4 teaspoons fresh lemon juice.
1/4 teaspoon salt
1/4 teaspoon freshly ground black pepper
2 tablespoons lightly roasted pine nuts

Set a wok over medium-high heat. Add the olive oil and turn to coat the inside of the pan. Add the garlic and stir-fry for 1 minute. Add the spinach and stir-fry until wilted. Remove the wok from the heat and add the lemon juice, salt, pepper, and pine nuts. Stir well and serve.

SQUASH AND SKILLET BEANS, 100 calories (4 servings)

1 ½ cups yellow squash sliced into 1/4-inch pieces (about 1 ½ medium)
1 ½ cups zucchini sliced into 1/4-inch pieces (about 1 ½ medium)
1 cup cubed pared Hubbard or acorn squash (about 4 ounces)
½ cup chopped onion (about 1 medium)
2 cans (16 ounces) kidney beans, drained
1 cup chicken broth
1 ½ tablespoons chopped jalapeno chili (about 1 small)
1 large garlic clove, finely chopped
1/4 cup snipped fresh cilantro

Heat all ingredients except cilantro to boiling in a 10-inch nonstick skillet and then reduce heat. Cover and simmer for 7 minutes. Stir in cilantro.

SQUASH AND ROASTED ZUCCHINI, 61 calories (4 servings)

1 tablespoon extra-virgin olive oil
3/4 pounds zucchini, sliced ½ inch thick (about 3 cups)
3/4 pounds yellow summer squash, sliced ½ inch thick (about 3 cups)
2 cloves garlic, minced
1 tablespoon chopped fresh rosemary, or ½ teaspoon dried rosemary, crushed
½ teaspoon kosher salt
½ teaspoon freshly ground black pepper

In a small saucepan, cook garlic in hot olive oil over medium heat for 1 minute. Stir in rosemary, pepper, and salt. Place zucchini and squash in a 13 x 9 x 2-inch baking pan and add oil mixture. Toss to coat and roast, uncovered, in a 425⁰ oven for 20 minutes, turning the vegetables once.

SUGAR SNAP PEAS WITH BASIL AND TOMATOES, 101 calories (4 servings)

2 teaspoons extra-virgin olive oil
3/4 pound sugar snap peas, strings removed
1 can (14 ½ ounces) stewed tomatoes, drained
3 cloves garlic, slivered
1/4 cup minced fresh basil
½ teaspoon salt

In a large nonstick skillet, heat the oil over medium heat, then add the garlic and cook for 1 minute. Add the other ingredients, stirring frequently, and cook for about 4 minutes.

BAKED TOFU CUTLETS, 108 calories (4 servings)

16 ounces firm tofu
4 tablespoons fresh lime juice
4 tablespoons soy sauce
1 teaspoon honey
1 teaspoon minced fresh gingerroot
1 teaspoon minced garlic
1 teaspoon chili sauce

Slice the tofu into 4 slices lengthwise. In a flat pan or nonstick baking dish just large enough to hold the slices in a single layer, combine remaining ingredients and then place the tofu in the marinade and refrigerate for 2-6 hours, turning occasionally. Bake in a preheated 350⁰ oven for 45 minutes.

TOFU TERIYAKI, 108 calories (3 servings)

2 tablespoons safflower oil
12 ounces silken extra-firm tofu

teriyake marinade
3 tablespoons low-sodium soy sauce
2 tablespoons freshly squeezed lemon juice
2 tablespoons honey
1 tablespoons dark sesame oil
2 teaspoon minced garlic
2 teaspoons minced gingeroot

Combine the ingredients for the marinade in a small bowl. Slice the tofu into bite-size pieces. Place the tofu in a square glass baking dish and cover with the marinade. Cover and marinate for 1 hour at room temperature, or 8 hours in the refrigerator. Heat the safflower oil in a nonstick skillet over medium-high heat. Transfer the tofu with a slotted spatula to the skillet and cook for 4 minutes. Use the extra marinade for dipping, if desired.

WARM TOMATO MOZZARELLA, 76 calories (2 serving)

vegetable cooking spray
1/4 teaspoon extra-virgin olive oil
8 slices tomato
1/4 teaspoon salt
4 garlic cloves, minced

4 tablespoons shredded low-fat mozzarella cheese
4 tablespoons grated Parmesan cheese
2 tablespoons finely chopped fresh parsley

Spray a nonstick baking pan with vegetable spray and place the tomato slices on the pan. Sprinkle salt on the tomatoes and broil for 3 minutes. Mix the olive oil, garlic, and cheese in a small bowl and spread over the tomato slices. Broil again for 4 minutes. Sprinkle with parsley and serve.

GARDEN-HARVEST VEGETABLES, 104 calories (3 servings)

vegetable cooking spray
1 cup sliced carrot (½-inch thick)
2 medium onions, each cut into 8 wedges
3 cups slices zucchini (1-inch thick)
2 cups broccoli florets
4 large mushrooms, quartered
2 garlic cloves, minced
1 tablespoon dried parsley flakes
1 teaspoon dried rosemary
1 teaspoon dried tarragon
1 teaspoon chicken-flavored bouillon granules
1/4 teaspoon salt
1/8 teaspoon freshly ground black pepper
1/4 cup water
1 teaspoon cornstarch

Place a large nonstick skillet coated with vegetable cooking spray over medium-high heat. Add carrots and onions and saute 8 minutes. Add zucchini and next 3 ingredients and saute 5 minutes. Add parsley and next 5 ingredients and saute 3 minutes. Combine water and cornstarch in a small bowl, add to skillet, and bring to a boil. Cook, stirring constantly, for 1 minute.

VEGETABLE KEBABS, 83 calories (4 servings)

1 large eggplant, cut in half and diced into 1-inch pieces
1 large green pepper, cut in half and cored and cut into 1-inch pieces
4 zucchini, sliced diagonally into 1-inch thick pieces
12 cherry tomatoes, with the tough cores removed
12 peeled pickling onions
12 button mushrooms, rinsed
4 tablespoons extra-virgin olive oil
2 ½ tablespoons lemon juice
3/4 teaspoon salt
1/4 teaspoon freshly ground black pepper

Put all the vegetables into a large bowl and pour in the remaining ingredients. Mix well and let stand covered with plastic wrap for 30 minutes, stirring occasionally. Thread the vegetables alternately onto skewers and brush with the marinade. Broil in a broiler pan for 4 minutes, turning frequently and basting with the marinade.

ASIAN VEGETABLE STIR-FRY, 102 calories (3 servings)

1 tablespoons vegetable oil
½ Vidalia or other sweet onion, cut into 4 wedges
1 small zucchini, quartered lengthwise and cut into 1-inch thick slices (about 2 cups)
1 small yellow squash, quartered lengthwise and cut into 1-inch thick slices (about 2 cups)
½ cup chopped celery
1 cups sliced green bell pepper (1/4-inch thick)
1/4 cup water
1/8 cup drained, sliced water chestnuts
1 cup thinly sliced napa (Chinese) cabbage
½ tablespoon pine nuts
1 tablespoon tomato paste
½ tablespoon rice vinegar
½ tablespoon low-sodium soy sauce
½ teaspoon curry powder
1/4 teaspoon salt
1/8 teaspoon freshly ground black pepper

Heat oil in a stir-fry pan or wok over medium heat. Add onion, stir-fry 1 minute. Increase heat to medium-high and add zucchini, yellow squash, and celery and stir-fry 5 minutes. Add bell-pepper, water, and water chestnuts, stir-fry 3 minutes. Combine last 6 ingredients in a small bowl and add to the vegetables. Bring to a boil, and cook 1 minute. Stir in cabbage and pine nuts and cook 30 seconds.

VEGETABLE CHILI, 110 calories (4 servings)

4 tablespoons vegetable stock
3 onions, chopped
1 carrot, chopped
1 15-ounce can red kidney beans, drained and rinsed
1 28-ounce can plus 1 14-ounce can tomatoes, chopped with their juice
1/3 cup fine or medium-grain bulgur
1 tablespoon minced jalapeno pepper (fresh or canned)
2 garlic cloves, minced
3 teaspoons chili powder
1 teaspoon ground cumin
1 teaspoon brown sugar

In a Dutch oven or a large saucepan, heat the vegetable stock over medium heat. Add the onion, carrot, pepper, garlic, chili powder, and cumin and braise, covered, for 6 minutes. Add the tomatoes with their juice and the sugar and cook for 5 minutes over high heat. Stir in the beans and bulgur, and reduce heat to low. Simmer uncovered for 15 minutes.

VEGETABLE STIR-FRY, 80 calories (3 servings)

1 ½ teaspoons canola oil
1 cup thinly sliced scallions
½ cup julienned carrot
1/4 pound asparagus, sliced 1/4 inch thick (4 spears)
1/4 pound fresh oyster mushrooms, sliced
½ cup thinly sliced red radish
½ teaspoon grated peeled fresh ginger
2 tablespoons vegetable stock
½ teaspoon salt
1/4 teaspoon freshly ground black pepper
1 tablespoon fresh lemon juice
4 cups small spinach leaves, well rinsed
2 teaspoons toasted sesame seeds

Set a wok over high heat. Add the oil and swirl to coat the inside of the pan. Add the scallions, carrot and ginger, and stir-fry briefly. Gradually add the asparagus, mushrooms, and radish while stirring. Slowly add the vegetable stock mixed with salt, pepper, and lemon juice. Toss well and serve over spinach. Sprinkle with sesame seeds.

VEGETABLE AND PASTA, 91 calories (4 servings)

½ cup packaged dried rotini pasta or elbow macaroni
3/4 cup broccoli flowerets
3/4 cup cauliflower flowerets
1 9-ounce package frozen artichoke hearts
½ cup sliced carrot
1/4 cup sliced green onions
½ cup reduced-calorie Italian dressing
Leaf lettuce slices if desired

Cook the pasta according to package directions, but omit any oil. Add the broccoli and cauliflower to boiling pasta for the last 1 minute of cooking. Drain and rinse with cold water. Drain well. Cook the artichoke hearts according to package directions. Drain and rinse with cold water. Drain well. Halve any large pieces. In a large mixing bowl, combine the two mixtures and add the carrots and green onions. Add the dressing and toss well. Cover and chill for 2-24 hours. Serve on lettuce-lined plates.

ZUCCHINI "PASTA" WITH MINT PESTO, 80 calories (4 servings)

vegetable cooking spray
2 teaspoons extra-virgin olive oil
3 yellow summer squashes (about 3/4 pounds) cut into long, narrow ribbons
3 zucchini (about 3/4 pound) cut into long, narrow ribbons
1 cup firmly packed fresh mint leaves
½ cup vegetable stock or broth
3 tablespoons grated asiago cheese
2 garlic cloves, cut up
½ cup chopped shallot
1 ½ teaspoon dried thyme
1/4 teaspoon salt
1/8 teaspoon freshly ground black pepper

Blend the mint, vegetable stock, cheese, garlic and olive oil until smooth. Heat a large nonstick frying pan over medium heat and coat the pan with vegetable cooking spray. Add the shallots and saute for 3 minutes. Add the yellow squash, zucchini, thyme and seasoning and saute 8 minutes. Stir in the mint pesto and heat for 1 minute. Serve hot.

STIR-FRIED ZUCCHINI AND SNOW PEAS, 80 calories (2 serving)

vegetable cooking spray
2 cup zucchini, cut into 1/4-inch slices
2 cup snow peas
4 tablespoons chopped leek
4 tablespoons water
1/4 teaspoon salt
½ teaspoon freshly ground black pepper

Heat a wok over high heat and spray with vegetable cooking spray. Add the zucchini, snow peas, and leek and stir for 2 minutes. Lower the heat to medium if the pan starts to smoke. Drizzle in the water and stir for 1 minute. Sprinkle with salt and pepper before serving, and mix well.

SOUPS

You can make your own fresh stock if desired, but during the initial phase of your diet, I recommend you buy store-bought stock for convenience. If you decide to add crackers, be sure to compute the calorie totals accordingly. 1 oyster cracker has 4 calories, 1 saltine cracker has 13 calories

SPICY BARLEY SOUP, 101 calories (4 servings)

½ tablespoon canola, safflower, or corn oil
1 large onions, finely chopped
1/2 large garlic clove, minced
4 medium-sized fresh mushrooms, sliced
4 cups vegetable stock, or 2 vegetarian bouillon packets (or cubes) reconstituted with 4 cups of water
½ large carrot, thinly sliced
1 large celery stalks, thinly sliced
1 ½ tablespoons reduced-sodium or regular tomato paste
½ cup turnip, peeled and dried
1/8 cup pearl barley
1/8 cup fresh parsley leaves, chopped
1 large bay leaf
½ teaspoon marjoram leaves
1/4 teaspoon dried thyme leaves
1/4 teaspoon powdered mustard
1/8 teaspoon celery seed
1/8 teaspoon freshly ground black pepper

In a large saucepan or small soup pot, combine oil, onions, garlic, mushrooms, and 3 tablespoons vegetable stock. Cook over medium heat, stirring frequently for 6 minutes, or until onions are tender. Add all remaining ingredients, stirring well, and bring mixture to a boil. Cover, lower heat, and simmer for 1 ½ hours. Skim the oil from the surface and discard.

BEET BORSCHT, 104 calories (4 servings)

vegetable cooking spray
2 medium beets, peeled, cut into julienne strips
1/4 tablespoon margarine
3 cups vegetable stock
½ small head red cabbage, thinly sliced, or shredded
1 carrot, cut into julienne strips
½ clove garlic, minced
1 bay leaf
1 teaspoon sugar
1 tablespoon cider vinegar
1/4 teaspoon salt

136

1/8 teaspoon freshly ground black pepper
4 ounces all vegetable-protein sausage style links

Saute beets in margarine in Dutch oven 3-4 minutes. Add next 9 ingredients and heat to boiling. Reduce heat and simmer, covered, for 25 minutes. Spray small skillet with vegetable cooking spray and heat over medium heat until hot. Cook sausage-style links over medium heat about 5 minutes, until brown on both sides. Cut links into 1-inch pieces and stir into soup. Cook 5 minutes. Sprinkle with dill weed or parsley, if desired.

CANNELLINI BEAN AND SPINACH SOUP, 100 calories (3 servings)

2 14 ½-ounce cans vegetable broth or reduced-sodium chicken broth
1 ½ cups water
1 15-ounce can white kidney beans or navy beans, rinsed and drained
2 cups coarsely chopped fresh spinach or ½ of a 10-ounce package frozen chopped spinach, thawed and drained
1/4 cup finely chopped onion
1/4 cup snipped fresh basil or 2 teaspoons dried basil, crushed
3 cloves garlic, minced
1 bay leaf
1 tablespoon diced pimento
½ teaspoon freshly ground black pepper

In a large sauce pan, combine the broth and water and bring to boiling. Stir in onion, basil, garlic, pepper, and bay leaf. Return to boiling, reduce heat, and simmer, covered, for 10 minutes. Stir in beans, spinach, and pimentos, and cook for 3 minutes. Discard bay leaf.

CREAM OF BROCCOLI SOUP, 99 calories (4 servings)

canola oil spray
½ cup chopped white onion
3 cups broccoli florets
½ cup chopped celery
1 ½ cups low-sodium vegetable broth
1 ½ cups plain soy milk
1/4 cup all-purpose unbleached flour
2 cloves garlic, minced
1/3 cup water

Spray the bottom of medium stockpot with canola oil and heat over medium heat. Cook the garlic and onion for 5 minutes. Add the broccoli and celery and stir. Add the vegetable broth, cover, and cook for 8 minutes. Transfer to a blender and process until pureed. Return the soup to the stockpot and add the soy milk. Simmer over low heat for 5 minutes. Combine the flour and water and mix until smooth. Add to the soup and stir. Simmer for 2 minutes.

CARROT SOUP, 94 calories (3 servings)

1 pound carrots, peeled and cut into thick slices (about 3 cups)
1 medium-sized onion, peeled and roughly chopped
1 medium-sized turnip, peeled and roughly chopped
2 cloves garlic, minced
3 cups vegetable stock
3/4 teaspoon dried thyme
1/4 teaspoon salt
1/4 teaspoon cayenne pepper

Put the vegetables, garlic and stock into a large saucepan and bring to a boil. Reduce heat and simmer covered for 20 minutes. Add the seasonings and simmer for 5 minutes. Allow to cool and blend in a food processor. Reheat, if desired. Garnish with sunflower seeds, if desired.

SPICY CARROT PEANUT SOUP, 95 calories (3 servings)

½ tablespoon canola or other vegetable oil
½ large onion, thinly sliced (about 1 cup)
1 pound carrots, peeled and thinly sliced (about 3 cups)
½ celery stalk, thinly sliced
½ teaspoon salt
½ teaspoon Chinese chili paste
3 cups water
1 tablespoon peanut butter
1 ½ tablespoon soy sauce
1 tablespoon fresh lime juice
lime wedges for garnish

In a soup pot on medium heat, warm the oil and add the next 5 ingredients. Saute on high heat for 5 minutes, stirring often. Add the water, cover, and bring to a boil. Lower the heat and simmer for 25 minutes. Stir in the other ingredients and puree in a blender. Reheat, if necessary. Serve with lime wedges.

MANHATTAN STYLE CLAM CHOWDER, 101 calories (5 servings)

2 teaspoons tub-style margarine
1 large onion, finely chopped
1 small clove garlic, minced
2 large celery stalks, including leaves, diced
2 6 ½-ounce cans chopped clams, including juice
½ large green pepper, diced

138

1 large potato, peeled and finely diced
1 16-ounce can tomatoes, crushed, juice reserved
1 bay leaf
1 teaspoon lemon juice
½ teaspoon dried thyme leaves
½ teaspoon sugar
1/4 teaspoon dried marjoram leaves
1/8 teaspoon freshly ground black pepper

In a large, heavy saucepan or Dutch oven, melt margarine and then add onion, garlic, and celery. Cook for 5 minutes, stirring frequently. Drain juice from the clams into a measuring cup and add enough water to make 1 3/4 cups of liquid. Add this to the pan, along with green pepper and potato and bring to a boil. Cover, lower heat, and simmer 10 minutes, stirring occasionally. Add the clams and all remaining ingredients, and break up the tomatoes with a spoon. Re-cover and bring to a boil and then lower heat and simmer about 5 minutes. Remove the bay leaf before serving.

CHILLED CUCUMBER SOUP, 80 calories per cup (4 servings)

2 cups chicken broth
2 cups skim milk
4 small cucumbers, peeled and chopped
1 small onion
2 cloves garlic, minced
½ teaspoon Kosher salt
1/4 teaspoon freshly ground black pepper
1 tablespoons chopped parsley or dill if desired

Place onion and garlic in a blender or food processor and puree until smooth. Add cucumbers and puree until smooth again. Pour puree into a large bowl and add broth, milk, pepper, and salt. Chill for two hours. When serving, sprinkle with fresh parsley or dill.

CUCUMBER YOGURT SOUP, 95 calories (3 servings)

½ tablespoon canola or other vegetable oil
3 cucumbers, peeled
1 cup plain low-fat yogurt
½ garlic clove, minced or pressed
1/8 cup coarsely chopped fresh chives
½ tablespoon chopped fresh dill
1 tablespoon chopped fresh mint or 1 teaspoon dried
1 teaspoon fresh lemon juice
1 teaspoon honey
½ teaspoon salt
1/8 teaspoon freshly ground black pepper

Coarsely chop two of the cucumbers and combine them in a medium bowl with the other ingredients. Puree in a blender until smooth. Seed and dice the remaining cucumber and add to the soup.

EGG DROP SOUP WITH CRABMEAT AND VEGETABLES, 108 calories (4 servings)

3 cups fat-free, low-sodium chicken broth
2 tablespoons cornstarch
4 ounces canned crabmeat, rinsed and drained
2 medium carrots, shredded
4 ounces snow peas, trimmed and cut into small strips
4 egg whites, lightly beaten
2 medium green onions, chopped
1 teaspoon toasted sesame oil
1/8 teaspoon salt
1/8 teaspoon freshly ground black pepper

In a medium saucepan, whisk together the broth and cornstarch. Bring to a simmer over medium-high heat, stirring occasionally, for 2 minutes. Stir in the carrots, snow peas, green onions, sesame oil, salt, and pepper. Simmer for 2 minutes. Stir in the crabmeat and simmer for 1 minute. Pour the egg whites in a thin, circular stream and gently stir until the egg whites resemble threads.

FENNEL AND LEMON SOUP, 75 calories (4 servings)

1 teaspoon extra-virgin olive oil
1 white onion, chopped
2 fennel bulbs, thinly sliced
2 ½ cups chicken stock
1 cup 2% milk
1 lemon, zested and juiced
1/4 teaspoon sea salt
1/8 teaspoon freshly ground black pepper

Heat a nonstick skill on high heat, and then add the olive oil. Reduce heat and add the onions and cook over low heat for 5 minutes. Stir in the fennel and then add the chicken stock and lemon zest and bring to a boil. Reduce heat, cover and simmer for 20 minutes. Transfer to a food processor and process until smooth. Add the milk, salt, pepper and lemon juice, and stir well.

GAZPACHO, 70 calories (makes 6 servings)

3 cups chopped, peeled tomatoes (about 4 large)
2 cups vegetable juice cocktail or low-sodium tomato juice

1/4 cup chopped fresh cilantro
½ cup chopped red bell peppers
½ cup chopped green bell peppers
½ cup diced Vidalia or other sweet onion
1 cup diced cucumber
1 cup shredded carrots
1/3 cup diced tomatillos
1/3 cup diced jicama
1/3 cup diced celery
1 teaspoon extra-virgin olive oil
1 tablespoon red wine vinegar
1 large clove garlic, minced
1 teaspoon Worcestershire sauce
½ teaspoon sea salt
1/4 teaspoon white pepper

To peel tomatoes, bring a large pot of water to a boil and prepare a bowl of ice water. Cut a small x on the bottom of each tomato and place them, a few at a time, into the boiled water. Allow to heat without boiling for 30 seconds, and then remove with a slotted spoon and transfer the tomatoes to ice water to cool. The skins should then slip off easily. Blend the tomatoes, olive oil, vinegar, Worcestershire sauce, cilantro, garlic, and yellow bell pepper in a large blender and then transfer to a mixing bowl and stir in the cucumber, red onion, tomatillos, jicama, celery, salt, and white pepper. Add the vegetable stock for proper consistency. Adjust the seasoning as desired. If you like your soup spicy, add 2-3 drops Tabasco or hot pepper sauce. Cover and chill before serving.

To increase the calorie intake of this soup to 100 calories, prepare 6 ounces of quick-cooking or instant couscous according to package instructions, and add to the soup before serving, stirring well. You may also add crackers, as described above.

SHRIMP GAZPACHO, 65 calories (6 servings)

2 teaspoons extra-virgin olive oil
2 cups tomato juice
3/4 teaspoon prepared horseradish
½ teaspoon chili powder
½ teaspoon salt
1/8 teaspoon dried thyme leaves
Pinch (generous) cayenne pepper
2 medium-large tomatoes, cored and finely chopped
1 medium-sized cucumber, peeled, seeded, and finely chopped
½ medium sweet green pepper, finely chopped
2 tablespoons scallions or chives, chopped
1 small clove garlic, minced
1 cup medium-sized deveined shrimp

In a medium-sized, non-corrosive bowl, stir together tomato juice and olive oil. Stir in next 5 ingredients and mix well. To cook the shrimp, place 1 pound in a quart of rapidly boiling water with 3 tablespoons of salt. Cover and return to a boil, then simmer 3-4 minutes for medium size shrimp, 5-7 minutes for large, and 7-8 minutes for jumbo. When cooked, the shrimp will no longer be glossy, and will be opaque in the center. Add the shrimp to the soup, along with the remainder of the ingredients, and stir well. Refrigerate covered for 4-12 hours before serving.

ORIENTAL HAM SOUP, 106 calories (4 servings)

4 cups water
1 ½ cups chopped bok choy
3/4 cup carrot cut into thin strips
3/4 cup chopped onion
2 tablespoons reduced-sodium soy sauce
Dash freshly ground black pepper
8 ounces lower-fat, lower-sodium cooked ham, cut into thin strips (about 1 ½ cups)
½ cup packaged dried regular or spinach noodles

In a large saucepan or Dutch oven, combine the first 6 ingredients. Bring to boiling and add the ham and noodles. Simmer, uncovered, for 10 minutes.

HOT AND SOUR SOUP, 105 calories per cup (4 servings)

1 tablespoon roasted sesame oil
4 cups of chicken or vegetable broth
4 ounces mushrooms, sliced
1 carrot, shredded
1/4 cup water chestnuts
2 cups chopped bok choy or spinach
2 cups broccoli florets
1 cup tofu
3 tablespoons dry white wine
2 tablespoons rice vinegar
2 tablespoons soy sauce
1 clove garlic, minced
½ - 1 teaspoon chili puree with garlic (to taste)

Warm the sesame oil in a large saucepan over medium heat and cook the garlic and mushrooms for several minutes. Stir in the other ingredients and bring to a boil. Reduce heat and simmer for at least 5 minutes. Adjust the seasoning if desired.

CURRIED LENTIL SOUP, 104 calories (3 servings)

1 teaspoon extra-virgin olive oil
½ cup chopped onion
½ cup sliced carrots
3/4 cup lentils
½ can (14.5 ounce) diced tomatoes, undrained
3 cups water
1 ½ teaspoon curry powder
1 tablespoon fresh basil or 1 teaspoons dried basil
½ teaspoon minced garlic
1/4 teaspoon salt
1/8 teaspoon freshly ground black pepper
garnish with fresh basil sprigs if desired

Heat olive oil in a large Dutch oven and add onion and saute for 4 minutes. Add curry powder and saute 1 minute. Add water, carrots, and lentils and bring to boil and then cover and reduce heat. Simmer for 40 minutes. Blend the mixture until smooth and then return to the Dutch oven and add the other ingredients and cook until thoroughly heated. If you use red lentils, simmer for 30 minutes instead of 40 minutes.

LENTIL-VEGETABLE SOUP, 91 calories (6 servings)

1 teaspoon extra-virgin olive oil
1 large onion, finely chopped
1 large celery stalk, diced
1 large carrot, diced
1 16-ounce can reduced-sodium stewed tomatoes or regular stewed tomatoes
½ cup red lentils, rinsed
½ large green pepper, diced
1 ½ cups small zucchini cubes
3 tablespoons long-grain white rice
2 cups water
1 large garlic clove, minced
2 cups chicken bouillon, reconstituted from cubes
½ teaspoon dried thyme leaves
1 bay leaf
½ teaspoon dried basil leaves
½ teaspoon sugar
1/4 teaspoon ground cumin
1/8 teaspoon freshly ground black pepper

In a Dutch oven or large, heavy pot, combine onion, celery, garlic, olive oil, and 3 tablespoons bouillon. Cook over medium heat, stirring frequently for 5 minutes. Add all the other ingredients and bring to a boil.

Lower heat and simmer 25 minutes, or until lentils are tender. Remove bay leaf before serving.

MISO NOODLE SOUP, 107 calories (5 servings)

1 teaspoon dark sesame oil
4 ounces somen or soba noodles
2 cans (14 ½ ounces) vegetable broth
8 fresh shiitake mushrooms, sliced 1/8-inch thick
1 cup chopped scallions
1 cup diagonally sliced carrot (1/8 inch thick)
1 teaspoon chile paste
1/4 cup white miso (soybean paste)
1 teaspoon peeled, minced fresh gingerroot
2 minced garlic clove

Cook the noodles according to the package directions, and then drain. Heat gingerroot and garlic in oil in a large saucepan over medium heat for 1 minute. Add broth and next 4 ingredients and bring to a boil and then reduce heat and simmer for 2 minutes uncovered. Stir in noodles and miso and cook for 1 minute.

SHRIMP MISO SOUP, 90 calories (2 servings)

1 teaspoon vegetable oil
2 green onions, including tops, finely chopped
1 garlic clove, minced
½ cup sliced mushrooms
½ teaspoon minced serrano chile
1 tablespoon red miso (soybean paste)
2 cups vegetable broth
1/4 cup small cooked, peeled shrimp

Heat oil in a saucepan over medium heat. Add onions, garlic, mushrooms, and chile, and cook for 7 minutes, stirring frequently. In a small bowl, dissolve miso in broth and add to the saucepan with the shrimp. Heat until hot, stirring occasionally, and be careful not to boil. To cook the shrimp, place 1 pound in a quart of rapidly boiling water with 3 tablespoons of salt. Cover and return to a boil, then simmer 3-4 minutes for medium size shrimp, 5-7 minutes for large, and 7-8 minutes for jumbo. When cooked, the shrimp will no longer be glossy, and will be opaque in the center. Add to the miso soup and stir while the soup is still hot.

MUSHROOM-BARLEY SOUP, 68 calories (4 servings)

3 1/4 cups low-sodium nonfat chicken broth
1/4 cup diced onion

144

1/4 cup diced celery
1/4 cup diced carrot
2 cloves garlic, minced
½ cup sliced white mushrooms
½ cup sliced shiitake mushrooms
1/8 cup barley
1 tablespoon sherry
1 tablespoon rice wine vinegar
1/8 cup skim milk
1 tablespoon chopped fresh scallions
1/4 teaspoon freshly ground black pepper

Heat 1/4 cup broth in a medium saucepan. Add onion, celery, and carrot and saute for 4 minutes. Add the garlic and saute for an additional 4 minutes. Add the mushrooms and saute for 4 more minutes. Stir in the barley and saute for 2 minutes. Add the remaining broth and bring to a boil. Reduce heat and simmer for 30 minutes. Stir in the remaining ingredients and heat through before serving.

PEA-AND-PASTA SOUP, 104 calories (4 servings)

4 cups (2 16-ounce cans) fat-free less-sodium chicken broth
1 cup frozen green peas
½ cup small uncooked pasta (such as pastina, orzo, or ditalini)
1 tablespoons chopped fresh parsley
2 tablespoons Riesling or other slightly sweet white wine
2 tablespoons grated fresh Parmesan cheese

Bring broth to a boil in a large saucepan over medium-high heat. Add peas, pasta, and parsley, reduce heat, and simmer 5 minutes, or until pasta is tender. Stir in wine and sprinkle with cheese.

CURRIED SPLIT PEA SOUP, 94 calories (4 servings)

4 cups vegetable stock
1 cup yellow split peas
½ cup minced onion
1 garlic clove, minced
½ teaspoon curry powder
1/4 teaspoon turmeric
½ tablespoon black peppercorns
6 whole cloves
½ bay leaf
½ teaspoon mustard seeds
1/4 cup nonfat plain yogurt
1 tablespoon lemon juice
1/4 teaspoon salt

1/8 teaspoon freshly ground black pepper
cilantro for garnish

In a large saucepan, combine the vegetable stock, peas, onion, garlic, curry powder, and turmeric. In a piece of cheesecloth, tie together the peppercorns, cloves, bay leaf, and mustard seeds, and add to the saucepan. Bring to a boil and then reduce the heat and simmer, covered, for 1 hour. Squeeze and then discard the spice bag. When the soup has cooled, process in a blender to a coarse puree. Return to the saucepan and heat through, stirring in the yogurt, lemon juice, salt and pepper. Garnish with cilantro when serving.

ROASTED RED BELL PEPPER SOUP, 106 calories (4 servings)

1 tablespoon extra-virgin olive oil
1 12-ounce jar of roasted red bell peppers
1 ½ cup mashed silken firm tofu (12 ounces)
1 1/4 cup vegetable stock
2 tablespoons red wine vinegar
2 teaspoons minced garlic
1 teaspoon sugar
1 tablespoon minced fresh thyme or 1 teaspoon dried thyme
1/4 teaspoon salt
½ teaspoon freshly ground black pepper

Put all the ingredients in a food processor, and process until smooth and creamy. Refrigerate in a covered container for at least 3 hours before serving chilled.

TWO-POTATO BISQUE, 100 calories (5 servings)

1 large sweet potato (yam), peeled and cut into 1-inch cubes
1 large baking potato, peeled and cut into 1-inch cubes
1 medium onion, chopped
2 cloves garlic, minced
1 bay leaf
½ teaspoon salt
1 teaspoon dried thyme leaves
2 cups canned fat-free broth
1 cup buttermilk
1 cup skim milk
2 tablespoons lime juice

In a large pot, combine the first 8 ingredients and bring to a boil. Reduce heat and simmer, covered, for 15 minutes. Pour into a food processor and blend to smooth. Return to pot and add the other 3 ingredients. Cook over low heat for 4 minutes. Remove bay leaf before serving.

POTATO VEGETABLE SOUP, 105 calories (5 servings)

½ pound (2 medium-size) waxy potatoes, peeled and diced
1 pound carrots, chopped
2 medium-size leeks, white part only, well washed and sliced
4 garlic cloves, minced
5 cups water
½ teaspoon salt
1/4 teaspoon freshly ground black pepper
½ cup 2% milk
2 bunches of cilantro, stems trimmed
cilantro leaves for garnish

Combine the first 7 ingredients in a large pot and bring to a boil. Reduce heat, cover, and simmer for 1 hour. Add the cilantro and pour into a food processor and blend to smooth. Return to the pot, add the milk, and heat through. Serve with cilantro leaves as garnish.

PUMPKIN SOUP, 85 calories (5 servings)

1 teaspoon extra-virgin olive oil
1 medium-sized onion, finely minced (about ½ cup)
2 celery stalks, finely chopped
1 medium-sized carrot, finely chopped
2 ½ cups canned fat-free chicken broth
2 tablespoons flour
1 15-ounce can solid-pack unsweetened pumpkin puree (not pie filling)
1 cup skim milk
1 teaspoon sugar
1/8 teaspoon ground ginger
1/8 teaspoon ground nutmeg
1/8 teaspoon ground cloves
1/8 teaspoon ground mace
1/4 teaspoon salt
1/8 teaspoon white pepper

In a large saucepan, heat the olive oil over medium heat. Add onion, celery, carrot, and 4 tablespoons of broth. Cook, stirring frequently, for 5 minutes. Add flour and stir to combine well and cook, stirring for 1 minute. Slowly add the remaining stock and then stir in the rest of the ingredients and bring to a boil. Lower heat and simmer, covered, for 20 minutes.

ORIENTAL SEAFOOD SOUP, 104 calories (6 servings)

1 small unpared cucumber
4 cups (2 16-ounce cans) chicken broth
1 tablespoon soy sauce

1/8 teaspoon ground ginger
dash of fresly ground black pepper
2 ounces uncooked vermicelli
½ pound firm lean fish fillets, cut into ½ inch slices
1 can (4 ½ ounces) tiny shrimp, rinsed and drained
5 cups torn spinach (about 4 ounces)
1/4 cup sliced green onions (with tops)

Cut cucumber lengthwise into halves, remove seeds and cut each half crosswise into thin slices. Heat chicken broth, water, soy sauce, ginger and pepper to boiling in 3-quart nonstick saucepan. Stir in vermicelli and heat to boiling. Cook uncovered for 4 minutes and stir in cucumber, fish and shrimp. Heat to boiling, reduce heat and simmer uncovered for 1 minute. Stir in spinach until wilted, about 1-2 minutes. Sprinkle each serving with green onions.

CURRIED BUTTERNUT SQUASH SOUP, 89 calories (4 servings)

2 cups chopped, peeled butternut squash
1 Granny Smith apple, peeled, cored, and chopped
1 medium onion, chopped
1 garlic clove, chopped
1 teaspoon curry powder
½ teaspoon ground cinnamon
2 cups water
1 cup unsweetened soy milk
1/8 teaspoon salt
1/8 teaspoon freshly ground black pepper

Combine the first 7 ingredients in a saucepan. Bring the liquid to a boil over medium-high heat, cover, and simmer for 25 minutes. Puree the soup in a blender, and then blend in the soy milk. Season with salt and pepper and serve.

FRESH TOMATO RICE SOUP, 100 calories (4 servings)

3 cups of chicken broth
1/4 cup of instant or parboiled long-grain white rice
1 medium onion, chopped
3 tomatoes, chopped, with juice
2 cloves of garlic, minced
½ teaspoon dried oregano
½ teaspoon freshly ground black pepper

Prepare rice by boiling in water and then draining. Place chicken broth in a large saucepan and add all the ingredients. Bring to a boil, reduce heat and simmer for 20 minutes. Sprinkle with Italian parsley if desired.

TOMATO SOUP WITH VERMICELLI, 104 calories (3 servings)

1 tablespoon extra-virgin olive oil
1 cup diced onions
1 ½ garlic cloves, minced or pressed
1/8 teaspoon cayenne pepper
½ teaspoon ground coriander
½ teaspoon ground cumin
1/4 teaspoon curry powder
1/4 teaspoon ground cinnamon
½ teaspoon salt
½ tablespoon freshly grated orange peel
1 ½ cups undrained canned tomatoes, chopped (½ 28-ounce can)
1 ½ cups vegetable stock
1 cup diced red bell peppers
1 cup thinly sliced celery
½ cup vermicelli, broken into ½-inch pieces
1 teaspoon fresh lemon juice

Heat the olive oil in a soup pot, add the onions and garlic, and saute on medium heat for 10 minutes. Add the next 7 ingredients and saute for 2 minutes, stirring constantly. Add the tomatoes and vegetable stock, cover, and bring to a boil. Add the peppers and celery, return the mixture to a boil, and cook for 5 minutes. Add the vermicelli and simmer, uncovered, for 5 minutes. Stir in the lemon juice and serve.

TOMATO-BASIL SOUP, 104 calories (4 servings)

2 cups chopped seeded peeled tomatoes (about 2 large)
2 cups low-sodium tomato juice
1/4 cup fresh basil leaves
½ cup 1% low-fat milk
1/8 teaspoon salt
1/8 teaspoon cracked black pepper
1/4 cup (2-ounces) ½-less-fat cream cheese, softened

Bring tomatoes and juice to a boil in a medium sauce pan. Reduce heat, simmer uncovered for 30 minutes. Place mixture and basil leaves in a blender and process until smooth. Return pureed mixture to pan, stir in milk, salt, pepper, and cream cheese with a whisk. Cook over medium heat about 5 minutes, or until thick. Garnish with sliced basil if desired.

CREAM OF TOMATO SOUP, 64 calories (3 servings)

½ tablespoon vegetable oil
½ medium onion, chopped
1 small carrot, chopped
1 celery stalk, chopped
1 garlic clove, minced
3 ripe tomatoes, chopped
3 crushed black peppercorns
1 bay leaf
2 cups vegetable stock
1 cup soy milk
1/4 teaspoon salt
1 teaspoon lime juice

Heat the oil in a medium pot over medium-high heat and saute the onion, carrot and celery for 7 minutes. Add the garlic and saute for 1 minute. Lower the heat and add the tomatoes, peppercorns, vegetable stock, salt, and lime juice and let the soup simmer for 35 minutes, stirring occasionally. Remove from heat and allow to cool slightly. Remove the bay leaf and puree the soup in a blender until smooth. Return soup to the pot and add the soy milk, heating thoroughly on low heat.

TOMATO BISQUE, 77 calories (4 servings)

4 cups peeled fresh tomatoes, or 2 (14 ½ -ounce) cans no-salt-added diced tomatoes
1 cup fat-free plain yogurt
1/4 teaspoon Tabasco sauce
2 large cloves garlic, crushed
1 1/4 teaspoon prepared horseradish
½ teaspoon salt
1/4 teaspoon freshly ground black pepper

Put all ingredients in a blender or food processor and puree until smooth. Serve chilled or at room temperature.

TURKEY BARLEY SOUP, 87 calories (4 servings)

6 cups water
1/4 cup barley
1 cup chopped onions
½ cup chopped celery
1 tablespoon chicken bouillon granules
½ pound turkey breast, boned, skinned and cut into bite-size pieces
1 teaspoon sour-cream-and-butter-flavored sprinkles
½ teaspoon salt-free lemon-pepper seasoning

1/8 teaspoon celery seed

Boil the water in a large saucepan over high heat. Add the barley and reduce the heat and simmer for 15 minutes, stirring occasionally. Add the onions, celery, and bouillon granules and continue cooking for 20 minutes. Add the other ingredients and cook for 20 minutes.

ZUCCHINI AND CHEDDAR CHEESE SOUP, 100 calories (4 servings)

3 cups reduced-sodium chicken broth
1 ½ pounds zucchini (about 3 medium), cut into 1-inch pieces
1 tablespoon chopped fresh tarragon or 1 teaspoon dried
½ cup shredded reduced-fat Cheddar cheese (2 ounces)
1/4 teaspoon salt
1/4 teaspoon freshly ground black pepper

Place broth, zucchini and tarragon in a medium saucepan and bring to a boil over high heat. Reduce to a simmer and cook uncovered for 8 minutes. Puree in a blender and return to the pan and heat over medium-high heat, slowly stirring in the cheese until it is incorporated. Add salt and pepper and serve hot or cold.

POTATOES

LARRY'S CELERY MASHED POTATOES, 100 calories (4 servings)

3 large potatoes, such as Yukon Gold, peeled and cut into small cubes
1/4 cup skim milk
1/4 cup soft tofu
1/4 cup water
2 medium garlic cloves, minced
2 tablespoons freshly grated, fat-free Parmesan cheese
5 celery stalks without leaves, minced
½ teaspoon salt
½ teaspoon freshly ground black pepper

In a 2-quart casserole, combine potatoes, water, and garlic. Cover
and Microwave at High for 14 minutes, stirring once after 7 minutes. Add
milk, tofu, salt, pepper, and cheese and beat or mash until desired texture. Add
celery, stir, and heat for 30 seconds in Microwave. Sprinkle paprika over top if
desired.

POTATO CRISPS, 75 calories (4 servings)

vegetable cooking spray
2 large potatoes, cut into 1/8 inch slices
1/4 teaspoon garlic powder
½ teaspoon salt
1/4 teaspoon pepper
1/2 teaspoon paprika
2 tablespoons chicken broth

Line a large baking sheet with aluminum foil. Spray the foil with
vegetable cooking spray. Arrange the potato slices on the baking sheet in a
single layer. Sprinkle with the garlic, paprika, salt, and pepper if desired.
Drizzle with chicken broth. Bake in a 450° oven for 20 minutes, or until the
potatoes are crisp.

ROASTED SWEET POTATO WEDGES, 101 calories (4 servings)

vegetable cooking spray
2 medium sweet potatoes, peeled
1 teaspoon extra-virgin olive oil
½ teaspoon curry powder
1/4 teaspoon ground cumin
1/8 teaspoon ground cloves
1/4 teaspoon salt
1/8 teaspoon freshly ground black pepper

Preheat oven to 425°. Cut the sweet potatoes in half lengthwise, then cut each half lengthwise into 4 wedges. Combine sweet potatoes, olive oil, and remaining ingredients in a bowl and toss gently to coat. Line a large baking sheet with aluminum foil and spray with vegetable cooking spray. Place potato wedges on the baking sheet and bake for 25 minutes.

HERBED POTATO WEDGES, 108 calories (4 servings)

vegetable cooking spray
2 medium baking potatoes
2 teaspoons extra-virgin olive oil
2 teaspoons balsamic vinegar
1 tablespoon grated Parmesan cheese
1 tablespoon Italian style fine dry bread crumbs (such as Contadina)
1/4 teaspoon garlic powder

Scrub potatoes with a soft vegetable brush under running water. Cut the potatoes in half lengthwise, then cut each half lengthwise into 4 wedges. Line a large baking sheet with aluminum foil and spray with vegetable cooking spray. Place potato wedges on the baking sheet, skin sides down. Mix olive oil and vinegar in a small bowl and brush the potatoes. Combine Parmesan cheese, bread crumbs, Italian seasoning, pepper, and garlic powder and coat the potatoes. Bake in a 425^0 oven for 20-25 minutes.

CRISP BAKED POTATO SKINS 90 calories (3 servings)

vegetable cooking spray
6 baking potatoes, scrubbed clean
3 tablespoon paprika
3 tablespoon chili powder
3 tablespoons roasted ground cumin
3 tablespoons ground coriander
1 teaspoon garlic powder
1 teaspoon onion powder
1 teaspoon cayenne pepper
½ teaspoon dried thyme leaves
½ teaspoon dried oregano leaves
½ teaspoon dried rosemary leaves

Slice potato and remove the pulp and place the skins, cut side up, on a baking sheet lined with aluminum foil and spray with vegetable cooking spray. Combine the herbs and spices and sprinkle over the skins and bake in the center of the oven for 30 minutes at 425°. Remove the pan from the oven and spray the skins with a fine mist of water and return to the oven for another 15 minutes.

TWICE-BAKED POTATOES, 97 calories (4 servings)

2 medium baking potatoes
½ cup fat-free ricotta cheese
1 tablespoon snipped fresh chives or thinly sliced green onion tops
½ teaspoon salt
1/4 teaspoon freshly ground black pepper
2 tablespoons skimmed milk
Paprika

Prick potatoes with a fork and bake in a 425⁰ oven for 30 minutes. Cool and cut in half lengthwise. Gently scoop pulp from each potato half and mash with a potato masher or electric mixer at low speed. Add the ingredients, except for milk and paprika, and beat until smooth. Add milk, 1 tablespoon at a time, and beat until fluffy. Spoon the mixture into the shells and sprinkle with paprika. Place on baking sheet, cover loosely with foil, and bake in a 425⁰ oven for 10 minutes. Uncover and bake for 5 more minutes.

SANDWICHES

GRILLED COTTAGE CHEESE AND TOMATO SANDWICH, 105 calories (1 serving)

1 slice five-grain bread
1/4 cup low-fat cottage cheese
2 tablespoons diced tomato
1/8 teaspoon thyme
1/8 teaspoon basil
1/8 teaspoon salt
1/8 teaspoon freshly ground black pepper

Preheat broiler. In a small bowl, blend cottage cheese with next 5 ingredients and spread mixture over bread. Set 4-6 inches from heat and broil 1-2 minutes.

MARINATED MUSHROOM SANDWICH, 110 calories (1 serving)

1 thin slice pumpernickel bread
2 large mushrooms (2 ounces)
1/4 cup Light French Dressing
1 tablespoon low-fat sour cream
2 strips red bell pepper

Trim off the ends of mushroom stems. Cut into thin slices and place in a small bowl. Add French dressing and toss gently. Let stand for 30 minutes. Arrange slices on bread and top with the sour cream and red bell pepper.

EGG AND VEGETABLE SALAD SANDWICH, 95 calories (4 servings)

4 thin slices black or pumpernickel bread
4 extra large eggs
1/3 cup grated carrot
1/3 cup celery, finely chopped
2 tablespoons chives, chopped
3 tablespoons pitted Sicilian-style green olives, chopped
1 tablespoon shallots, finely chopped
1 tablespoon plain low-fat yogurt
1 tablespoon reduced-fat mayonnaise
1 teaspoon Dijon mustard
1/8 teaspoon freshly ground black pepper
2 cups fresh baby spinach
8 cherry or rape tomatoes

Place eggs in medium pot and add water to cover by 1 inch. Bring water to a full boil over medium heat and boil for 1 minute. Turn off the heat and cover the pot for 15 minutes. Drain the eggs, and run over cold water for 3 minutes. Peel the eggs and place 3 in a mixing bowl. Add the white from the fourth egg to the bowl. Chop the eggs and then add the next 9 ingredients. Mix with a fork until well combined. Place a slice of bread on a plate, and cover with 1/4 of the spinach. Mound 1/4 of the egg salad on top of the spinach and add 2 of the tomatoes, sliced, and serve.

TOFU AND VEGETABLE SALAD SANDWICH, 100 calories (4 servings)

4 thin slices black or pumpernickel bread
1 10-ounce package firm tofu, drained and crumbled
1/4 cup finely chopped carrot
2 tablespoons finely chopped green or red bell pepper
1/4 cup finely chopped celery
2 tablespoons finely chopped scallions
1 ½ tablespoon soy mayonnaise
2 teaspoons vinegar
1 teaspoon tumeric
½ teaspoon salt
½ teaspoon freshly ground black pepper
1 teaspoon hot sauce
1 teaspoon Dijon mustard
2 cups fresh baby spinach
8 cherry or rape tomatoes

Combine the tofu, carrot, bell pepper, celery and scallions in a large bowl. In a small bowl combine the next 7 ingredients, and mix well. Add the dressing to the tofu mixture and toss to coat. Place a slice of bread on a plate, and cover with 1/4 of the spinach. Mound 1/4 of the tofu salad on top of the spinach and add 2 of the tomatoes, sliced, and serve.

TUNA ROLL-UPS, 100 calories (4 servings)

4 slices low-calorie whole-wheat bread
1 can (6-ounce) solid white tuna
½ cup diced celery
2 tablespoons reduced-calorie spoonable salad dressing, such as Miracle Whip Light
1 teaspoon lemon juice
1/4 teaspoon dillweed

Combine tuna and diced celery in a bowl and toss gently. Add the dressing, lemon juice, and dillweed, and stir well. Spread mixture over each slice of bread.

COLD CUT OPEN-FACED SANDWICH, 85 calories (1 serving)

Herbert Shelton, the originator of the concept of *Natural Hygiene*, cautioned against eating sandwiches which combined bread and meat, based upon his belief that the process of digestion differed between primary food substances,[164] but I do not believe this is a significant problem in most people, and certainly should not affect you while you are on a reduced-calorie diet. You can choose your own spreads or meat for this sandwich, using 1 thin slice of bread with 1 teaspoon of mustard or calorie-reduced mayonnaise spread on top, and 1 slice of meat, such as chicken bologna, turkey bologna, chicken breast, ham, pork olive loaf, roast beef, salami, or turkey breast, and 1 slice of dill pickle.

MEAT AND FOWL ENTREES

You can make tasty meat and fowl entrees for only 100 calories, but you must be careful to only use the small portions prescribed. If you cannot do this in Stage II, wait until Stage III, when you can eat a double portion.

BLACKENED CHICKEN BREAST, 100 calories per serving (4 servings)

vegetable cooking spray
4 small chicken breasts (3-ounces), skinned and boned
1 teaspoon thyme
1 teaspoon basil
1/4 teaspoon Cayenne pepper
½ teaspoon paprika
½ teaspoon cumin
1/4 teaspoon salt
1/4 teaspoon freshly ground black pepper

Combine the seasonings on a small plate and roll each breast, coating both sides. Either spray a grill or cast-iron skillet with vegetable cooking spray. Pre-heat cooking surface on high heat for 15 minutes. Cook chicken for 5 minutes, and then turn to other side for 5 more minutes. Use exhaust fan to clear the fumes from the air if you are cooking inside.

TANDOORI CHICKEN, 110 calories (4 servings)

vegetable cooking spray
4 small chicken breasts (3-ounces), skinned and boned
3/4 cup coarsely chopped onion
1 teaspoon coarsely chopped peeled fresh ginger
2 garlic cloves, peeled
½ cup plain low-fat yogurt
1 tablespoon fresh lemon juice
1 teaspoon paprika
1 teaspoon ground cumin
1 teaspoon ground coriander seeds
½ teaspoon chili pepper
½ teaspoon salt
1/4 teaspoon freshly ground black pepper

Place the onion, ginger and garlic in a food processor, and process until finely chopped. Add the next 8 ingredients and pulse four times, or until blended. Make 3 diagonal cuts 1/4 inch deep across top of each chicken breast and combine the chicken and yogurt mixture in a large zip-top bag. Seal and marinate in refrigerator for 8 hours, turning occasionally. Remove chicken breasts and place on grill rack or broiler pan coated with vegetable cooking spray and cook 5 minutes on each side.

HOT-AND-SPICY ASIAN-RUBBED CHICKEN, 100 calories (4 servings)

vegetable cooking spray
4 small chicken breasts (3-ounces), skinned and boned
2 teaspoons five-spice powder
1 teaspoon sugar
½ teaspoon salt
½ teaspoon garlic powder
1/4 teaspoon freshly ground red pepper

      Combine the seasonings in a large bowl and then rub the chicken with the mixture. Place chicken on grill rack or broiler pan coated with vegetable cooking spray and grill 5 minutes on each side.

CHICKEN MARSALA, 110 calories (4 servings)

vegetable cooking spray
4 small chicken breasts (3-ounces), skinned and boned
1 ½ cups sliced fresh mushrooms
2 tablespoons sliced green onion
2 tablespoons water
1/4 teaspoon salt
1/4 cup dry Marsala or dry sherry

      Place the chicken breasts between 2 pieces of plastic wrap and pound lightly with the flat side of a meat mallet to about 1/4 inch thickness, working from the center to the edges. Spray an unheated large skillet with vegetable cooking spray and preheat over medium heat. Add chicken and cook for 6 minutes, turning to brown evenly. Remove chicken from the skillet and place each breast on a plate. Add the next 4 ingredients to the skillet, and cook over medium heat for 3 minutes. Add the wine and heat through. Spoon the mixture on the chicken breasts and serve.

GARLIC ROASTED GINGER CHICKEN, 100 calories (4 servings)

vegetable cooking spray
4 small chicken breasts (3-ounces), skinned and boned
1 tablespoon lemon juice
1 teaspoon extra-virgin olive oil
3 cloves garlic, minced
1 teaspoon grated fresh ginger
½ teaspoon ground sage
½ teaspoon seasoned salt

      Preheat oven to 425°. Place chicken, skin side up, on a roasting pan sprayed with vegetable cooking spray. In a small bowl, combine the other

159

ingredients and brush on the chicken breast halves. Bake for 35 minutes, and garnish with lemon slices and sage if desired.

LEMON-ROSEMARY CHICKEN BREASTS, 110 calories (4 servings)

4 small chicken breasts (3-ounces), skinned and boned
2 lemons
1 tablespoon chopped fresh rosemary or ½ teaspoon dried rosemary
1 garlic clove, finely chopped
2 tablespoons extra-virgin olive oil
½ teaspoon salt
1/4 teaspoon coarsely ground black pepper

Grate 2 teaspoons of peel from 1 lemon, and then cut thin slices from ½ lemon to use as garnish. Squeeze juice from remaining lemon into a medium bowl and stir in lemon peel, and next 5 ingredients. Add chicken breast halves to bowl and coat with the lemon-juice mixture. Grill chicken over medium heat for 5 minutes, brushing with remaining mixture. Turn chicken and grill for another 5 minutes. Garnish with lemon slices.

CHICKEN THIGHS WITH LEMON SAUCE, 111 calories (4 servings)

4 skinless chicken thighs (7-ounces)
3-4 tablespoons water
2 tablespoons lemon juice
1 tablespoon Worcestershire sauce
2 teaspoons extra-virgin olive oil
1 ½ teaspoon Dijon mustard
1/4 teaspoon salt
1/4 teaspoon freshly ground black pepper
1/4 cup chicken broth

Preheat the oven to 375^0. In a small bowl, mix the lemon juice, Worcestershire sauce, olive oil, mustard, salt, pepper, and 2 tablespoons of the water. Place the chicken in an oven-safe skillet and pour the mixture evenly over the top. Bake for 25 minutes, adding 1-2 tablespoons of water as necessary. Remove the chicken to a platter and keep warm. Add the broth to the skillet and cook over medium heat for 3 minutes. Spoon over the chicken and serve.

CRUNCHY DRUMSTICKS, 101 calories (4 servings)

4 chicken drumsticks
1/4 cup chicken stock
1/4 cup shredded wheat minibiscuits, crushed
1/4 teaspoon cayenne pepper

Dip the drumsticks in the chicken stock, and then roll them in the crushed biscuits mixed with the cayenne pepper. Bake for 30 minutes at 425° in a pre-heated oven.

TURKEY AND APPLE SAUSAGE, 110 calories (4 servings)

vegetable cooking spray
12 ounces turkey, without skin
2 tablespoons soft bread crumbs
½ cup shredded peeled apple
1 ½ teaspoons snipped fresh sage or ½ teaspoon dried sage, crushed
1/8 teaspoon paprika
1/4 teaspoon salt
1/4 teaspoon freshly ground red pepper

In a large bowl, combine bread crumbs, apple, sage, pepper, salt, and paprika. Add turkey and mix well. Shape mixture into 4 patties. Spray the unheated rack of a broiler pan with the vegetable cooking spray and arrange patties on the rack. Broil 4-5 inches from the heat for 5 minutes, turn and broil for another 5 minutes.

TURKEY PATTIES WITH CAJUN SAUCE, 100 calories (4 servings)

vegetable cooking spray
12 ounces ground turkey, without skin
1 tablespoon minced fresh onion
1 teaspoon paprika
1/4 teaspoon salt
1/4 teaspoon freshly ground red pepper
½ teaspoon chili powder
1 cup finely chopped onion
½ cup finely chopped green bell pepper
½ cup finely chopped celery
½ teaspoon cornstarch
1 cup chicken stock
1 teaspoon low-sodium Worcestershire sauce
1 teaspoon low-sodium soy sauce

In a large bowl, mix the turkey and next 5 ingredients, and then shape to form 4 patties. Spray the inside of a medium skillet with vegetable cooking spray and place over high heat. Add the turkey patties for 8 minutes, turning often with a spatula. Remove the patties and spray the skillet again with vegetable cooking spray. Add the onions, bell pepper, and celery, and saute over high heat for 5 minutes, stirring frequently. Dissolve the cornstarch in the stock and add to the skillet, cooking for 10 minutes. Spoon the sauce over each patty on individual plates.

TURKEY PORCUPINES, 110 calories (4 servings)

vegetable cooking spray
12 ounces ground turkey, without skin
1 cups broccoli slaw (found in the bagged salad section of the grocery)
1/4 cup soy protein (not soy flour)
1 tablespoon fresh lime juice
½ teaspoon Sweet & Slender, or 2 packets of Equal
½ teaspoon ginger
½ teaspoon lemon pepper
1 teaspoon seasoning salt
½ cup water

In a large mixing bowl, combine all of the ingredients and mix well. Form the mixture into 4 patties, and gently place them into a large skillet with a well-fitting lid and coated with vegetable cooking spray. Cover and cook for 10 minutes over medium heat. Turn the meatballs, cover and cook for another 5 minutes.

GRILLED VEAL OR PORK CHOPS, 113 calories (4 servings)

4 boneless veal loin chops or pork loin chops (3-ounces each)
1/3 cup red wine vinegar
1 tablespoon honey
2 teaspoons Worcestershire sauce
2 teaspoons Dijon mustard
1 ½ teaspoons snipped fresh thyme or ½ teaspoon dried thyme, crushed
1/4 teaspoon freshly ground black pepper

Place the chops in a plastic bag set in a deep bowl. Pour the remaining ingredients in a small bowl and stir well. Add the marinade mixture to the bag and marinate at room temperature for 30 minutes, occasionally turning the bag to mix well. Place the chops on a grill, or broil 5 inches from the heat, for 5 minutes. Brush the chops with the remaining marinade mixture and cook for 5 more minutes.

FISH ENTREES

PLAIN GRILLED FISH WITH SEASONING OF YOUR CHOICE

A dinner of plain grilled seafood is an excellent source of protein, with cooked and seasoned 3-ounce portions averaging 105 calories for striped or sea bass, 89 calories for cod, 93 calories for dolphinfish, 100 calories for grouper, 95 calories for haddock, 119 calories for halibut, 82 calories for monkfish, 103 calories for perch, 75 calories for orange roughy, 127 calories for salmon, 109 calories for snapper, 99 calories for sole (flounder), 157 calories for fresh tuna, 70 calories for canned chunk tuna, 101 calories for walleye pike, 82 calories for Alaska king crab, 83 calories for lobster tails, 75 calories for scallops, and 90 calories for shrimp (12 large). Feel free to grill your favorites with seasoning to your taste, but here are some delectable alternatives to choose from.

SMOKY CATFISH, 90 calories (4 servings)

vegetable cooking spray
12 ounces catfish or medium-fat fish fillets cut in 3-ounce portions
2 tablespoons lemon juice
1 tablespoon soy sauce
1 ½ teaspoons liquid smoke
1 clove garlic, finely chopped
1 tablespoon snipped fresh chives

Arrange fillets in rectangular baking dish, 12 x 7 ½ x 2 inches, sprayed with vegetable cooking spray. Mix remaining ingredients except chives and brush over fish. Cover and refrigerate about 30 minutes, brushing twice more. Bake uncovered in oven heated to 400⁰ for 20 minutes. Sprinkle with chives. You can also microwave for 3 minutes, rotate dish ½ turn, and microwave another 4 minutes.

COD AND SWEET PEPPERS, 116 calories (4 servings)

1 pound fresh cod cut in 4-ounce portions
3/4 cup chicken broth
1 medium onion, sliced and separated into rings
2 1/4 teaspoons snipped fresh oregano or marjoram or 3/4 teaspoon dried oregano or marjoram, crushed
½ teaspoon finely shredded lemon peel
1 tablespoon lemon juice
1 clove garlic, minced
1 ½ cups bite-sized strips green and/or red sweet peppers (2 small)

Rinse fish and pat dry. In a large skillet, combine broth, onion, oregano, lemon peel, lemon juice and garlic. Bring to a boil and reduce heat.

Simmer, covered, for 3 minutes. Place the fish fillets in the skillet and add sweet peppers. Cook covered, over medium heat, for 8 minutes, or until fish flakes when tested with a fork.

BAKED FLOUNDER, 105 calories (4 servings)

vegetable cooking spray
1 pound flounder fillets cut in 4-ounce portions
1 ½ cups vegetable juice
1 1/4 teaspoons lemon juice
½ cup diced onions
½ teaspoon garlic, minced
1/8 teaspoon freshly ground black pepper

Preheat oven to 375^0. Rinse fillets and pat dry and place in a shallow baking dish sprayed with vegetable cooking spray. Combine the remaining ingredients in a small saucepan and bring to a boil. Pour sauce over fish and bake for 20 minutes, basting occasionally.

SPICY HALIBUT, 102 calories (4 servings)

vegetable cooking spray
12 ounces halibut cut in 3-ounce portions.
1 tablespoon lime juice
1 tablespoon water
1 teaspoon paprika
1/4 teaspoon ground ginger
1/4 teaspoon ground allspice
½ teaspoon salt
1/4 teaspoon freshly ground black pepper

Brush fish with mixture of lime juice and water. In a small bowl, combine next 5 ingredients and rub onto fish. Arrange fish in a shallow baking pan sprayed with vegetable cooking spray and bake, uncovered, in a 450^0 oven for 10 minutes. Brush fish with pan juices and serve, if desired, garnished with lime wedges or lime peel strips.

MEDITERRANEAN HALIBUT, 102 calories (4 servings)

vegetable cooking spray
12 ounces halibut cut in 3-ounce portions
1 tablespoon extra-virgin olive oil
2 tablespoons lemon juice
1 tablespoon chopped onion
1 tablespoon coarsely chopped pimiento-stuffed olives
1 tablespoon capers

Place fish in square baking dish, 8 x 8 x 2 inches, sprayed with vegetable cooking spray. Mix remaining ingredients and spread over fish. Cover and refrigerate for 1 hour, turning once. Heat oven to 350^0. Cover and bake for 30 minutes.

SMOKED MONKFISH, 101 calories (4 servings)

1 tablespoon vegetable oil
12 ounces monkfish, cleaned and cut in 2-inch chunks
1 teaspoon five-spice powder
1 red onion, finely chopped
1-inch cube fresh root ginger, peeled and chopped
3 garlic cloves, crushed
½ teaspoon chili powder
2 teaspoons tomato puree
1 tablespoon lemon juice
2 tablespoons finely chopped fresh cilantro leaves

Heat the oil in a small saucepan over low to medium heat and add the five-spice powder and onions. Mix and fry for 5 minutes. Add the ginger, garlic and chile powder and cook for a further 1 minute. Add the tomato puree and stir before adding the monkfish. Cook the fish mixture for 7 minutes, stirring occasionally. Stir in the lemon juice and cilantro leaves before serving.

BROILED ORANGE ROUGHY, 92 calories (4 servings)

vegetable cooking spray
12 ounces orange roughy fillets cut in 3-ounce portions
3 tablespoons lemon juice
1 tablespoon Dijon mustard
1 tablespoon margarine, melted
1/4 teaspoon coarsely ground black pepper

Combine last 4 ingredients in a small bowl and stir well. Place fish on rack of a broiler pan coated with vegetable cooking spray. Brush with half of the lemon juice mixture. Broil 6 inches from heat with oven door partially opened for 5 minutes. Drizzle with the remaining lemon juice mixture.

LETTUCE-WRAPPED PERCH FILLETS, 105 calories (4 servings)

1 pound ocean perch fillets cut in 4-ounce portions
1 cup bottled clam juice
1 bay leaf
1/4 teaspoon thyme
4 large Boston lettuce leaves
1 carrot, cut into thin slices
2 celery stalks, cut into thin slices

1/4 teaspoon salt
1/8 teaspoon freshly ground black pepper

In a small saucepan, bring clam juice, bay leaf, and thyme to a boil over medium heat. Add lettuce leaves and boil 1 minute. Remove lettuce and spread on paper towel to drain. Add carrots and celery to hot broth and cook for 5 minutes. Place a fish fillet on each lettuce leave and divide the carrots and celery slices evenly over each fillet. Season with salt and pepper and fold over sides of each lettuce leaf, enclosing the fish completely. Put fish packages, seam side down, in a medium saucepan and pour the broth over the fish. Cover the saucepan and bring to a simmer, cooking for 7 minutes.

ZESTY RED SNAPPER WITH MUSHROOMS, 100 calories (4 servings)

vegetable cooking spray
12 ounces red snapper or lean fish fillets cut in 3-ounce portions
½ teaspoon paprika
1 ½ teaspoon snipped fresh tarragon leaves or ½ teaspoon dried tarragon leaves
1 ½ teaspoon snipped fresh oregano leaves or ½ teaspoon dried oregano leaves
½ teaspoon salt
1/8 teaspoon freshly ground red pepper
2 tablespoons lemon juice
1 cup sliced mushrooms (about 3-ounces)

Preheat oven to 425°. Place fish fillets in rectangular baking dish, 12 x 7 ½ x 2 inches, sprayed with vegetable cooking spray and brush with 1 tablespoon of the lemon juice. Mix paprika, tarragon, oregano, salt, and red pepper and rub both sides of the fish with herb mixture. Cook mushrooms in a 10-inch nonstick skillet sprayed with vegetable cooking spray over medium heat for 2 minutes, stirring occasionally. Place mushrooms over fish, cover and bake for 15-20 minutes.

BAKED RED SNAPPER CHINOISE, 96 calories (4 servings)

vegetable cooking spray
12 ounces red snapper fillets cut in 3-ounce portions
1 tablespoon light soy sauce
½ garlic clove, finely chopped
1 teaspoon finely chopped fresh ginger
½ cup vegetable broth
1 teaspoon sugar

Preheat oven to 425°. Combine last 5 ingredients in a shallow casserole sprayed with vegetable cooking spray and arrange snapper fillets in a single layer. Bake 15 minutes, basting with the sauce twice.

GRILLED ATLANTIC KING SALMON, 118 calories (4 servings)

1 pound salmon fillets cut in 4-ounce portions
1 teaspoon fresh dill
½ teaspoon salt
1/4 teaspoon freshly ground black pepper
fresh lemon wedges

Preheat grill to 400^0. Place the salmon fillets on the grill with the skin side down. Season with seasonings, and squeeze lemon onto each fillet. Close grill and turn heat down to medium low. Cook for 20 minutes.

LEMONY STEAMED SCROD, 99 calories (4 servings)

vegetable cooking spray
1 pound scrod fillets cut in 4-ounce portions
1 small onion, finely chopped
1/4 cup chopped parsley
1 teaspoon dill weed
1 teaspoon paprika
1 tablespoon lemon juice.
1/4 teaspoon salt
1/8 teaspoon freshly ground black pepper

Preheat oven to 400^0. Center each fillet on a 12-inch square of aluminum foil. Sprinkle with the remaining ingredients and fold foil over each fillet to make a packet. Be sure to pleat the seams and securely seal. Place on a baking sheet sprayed with vegetable cooking spray and bake for 30 minutes.

BROILED SOLE WITH LEMON, 96 calories (4 servings)

vegetable cooking spray
12 ounces sole fillets cut in 3-ounce portions
1 lemon, peeled and cut into 8 thin slices
2 tablespoons reduced-calorie mayonnaise
1 tablespoon Dijon mustard

Preheat oven to 425°. In a flameproof baking dish sprayed with vegetable cooking spray, arrange 4 groups of 2 lemon slices. Place 1 sole fillet on each pair of lemon slices. Combine mayonnaise and mustard and mix to blend well. Spread 2 teaspoons of the mixture over each fish fillet. Broil fish 4-6 inches from heat for 5 minutes, or until topping is bubbly and brown.

SAVORY BAKED SOLE, 100 calories (4 servings)

1 pound sole fillets cut in 4-ounce portions
½ cup chopped celery

1/4 teaspoon rosemary
1/4 teaspoon paprika
1 cup chopped tomatoes, well drained
½ cup chopped green onions
1/8 cup dry white wine
1/4 teaspoon salt
1/8 teaspoon freshly ground black pepper

Preheat oven to 400°. Sprinkle celery in a shallow baking pan. Arrange fish over the celery and sprinkle with salt, rosemary, pepper, and paprika. Top with tomatoes, onion and wine. Bake for 20 minutes. You can also heat in microwave on high power for 10 minutes.

MUSTARD SWORDFISH STEAKS, 100 calories (4 servings)

12 ounces swordfish steaks cut in 3-ounce portions
1 garlic clove, minced
2 tablespoons lemon juice
2 egg whites
2 tablespoons Dijon mustard
2 tablespoons chopped green onions (with tops)
1/4 teaspoon salt
1/8 teaspoon pepper

Place fish steaks on rack sprayed with nonstick cooking spray in a broiler pan. Mix lemon juice, salt, pepper, and garlic, and brush on top of the fish steaks. Broil with oven control set to broil with tops about 4 inches from heat for 5 minutes. Turn, brush with remaining lemon juice, and broil for another 3-5 minutes. Beat egg whites and fold in mustard and onions and spread mixture over fish. Broil for another 1 ½ minutes.

CITRUS TILAPIA, 95 calories (4 servings)

vegetable cooking spray
1 pound tilapia fillets cut in 4-ounce portions
½ teaspoon grated orange rind
1/4 cup unsweetened orange juice
½ teaspoon grated lime rind
2 tablespoons fresh lime juice
½ teaspoon ground cumin
1/4 teaspoon ground coriander
1/4 teaspoon hot sauce
½ teaspoon salt

Place fillets in a large shallow dish. In a small bowl, combine the rest of the ingredients and stir well. Pour over the fillets, cover, and leave in refrigerator for 2 hours. Remove fillets and preserve the marinade. Place fillets on a rack in a broiler pan coated with cooking spray. Broil 5 ½ inches from heat for 5 minutes on each side, basting frequently with the marinade.

FRESH TUNA CAKES, 115 calories per cake (4 servings)

vegetable cooking spray
12 ounces tuna cut into cubes and minced
1 ½ scallions, finely chopped
1 clove garlic, minced
2 tablespoons chopped freshly parsley
1 tablespoon sesame seeds
1 teaspoon grated fresh ginger
1 tablespoon rice wine
1 tablespoon reduced-sodium soy sauce
3 tablespoons dry whole grain breadcrumbs
1 tablespoon peanut or sesame oil

Combine the ingredients except for the breadcrumbs and oil in a medium bowl, and gently fold the mixture until you have a homogenous blend. Prepare 4 cakes, and then press each cake into the breadcrumbs. Warm the oil over medium-high heat in a medium nonstick skillet sprayed with vegetable cooking spray, and cook the cakes for 3 minutes on each side.

SPICY LEMON WALLEYE PIKE, 103 calories (4 servings)

vegetable cooking spray
1 pound walleye pike fillets cut in 4-ounce portions
2 tablespoons sugar
2 tablespoons lemon juice
1 teaspoon Worcestershire sauce
½ teaspoon paprika
1/4 teaspoon sea salt
½ teaspoon lemon pepper

Spray a pan with vegetable cooking spray and place in fillets which have been rinsed and patted dry. Mix the other ingredients in a small bowl and brush the fillets. Broil, turning and basting, for 10-15 minutes, until the fillets are flaky.

SHELLFISH DISHES

BAY SCALLOPS IN GINGER SAUCE, 100 calories (serves 4)

1 pound bay scallops
1 bunch watercress (2-3 ounces)
2 ½ tablespoons chicken broth
1 medium onion, finely chopped
1 ½ teaspoons minced fresh ginger
½ medium yellow bell pepper, finely chopped (½ cup)
1/8 teaspoon Kosher salt

   Wash watercress. Pat dry and chop. In a small saucepan, combine chicken broth, onion, ginger, and yellow pepper. Cook over medium heat 4 minutes, until onion is softened. Add watercress and salt. Cook, stirring occasionally, for 1-2 minutes. Stir in scallops and cook, stirring frequently, for 4 minutes, or until scallops are opaque.

SCALLOP AND SHRIMP KABOB, 110 calories (4 servings)

8 ounces fresh or frozen scallops, thoroughly rinsed
12 large fresh or frozen shrimp, peeled and deveined
12 fresh pea pods
1 orange cut into 8 wedges
1 garlic clove, minced
½ cup orange juice
1 teaspoon finely grated orange peel
2 tablespoons soy sauce
1 teaspoon grated peeled fresh gingerroot
1/4 teaspoon cayenne pepper

   Combine the last 6 ingredients in a plastic food-storage bag set in a deep bowl. Add the scallops and shrimp to the marinade and seal the bag. Turn and squeeze the bag to coat the seafood and marinate in the refrigerator for 30 minutes. Cook the pea pods in boiling water for 2 minutes. Wrap 1 pea pod around each shrimp and alternately thread them onto four 10-inch skewers with the scallops and orange wedges. Grill on an uncovered grill for 6 minutes. Turn and brush with the leftover marinade and grill for 6 minutes more. As an alternate, you can broil 4 inches from the heat in the same manner for 5 minutes on each side.

GRILLED SCALLOP AND TOMATO KABOBS, 123 calories (4 servings)

vegetable cooking spray
1 pound fresh sea scallops
20 cherry tomatoes
2 tablespoons low-sodium teriyaki sauce

Place scallops and tomatoes alternatively on 4 (12-inch) skewers and brush with 1 tablespoon teriyaki sauce. Coat grill rack with vegetable cooking spray and preheat to medium-hot. Place kabobs on rack and grill, uncovered, for 5 minutes. Turn kabobs and brush with remaining teriyaki sauce. Grill 10 minutes, or until scallops are opaque.

MEXICAN-STYLE GRILLED SHRIMP, 109 calories (4 servings)

vegetable cooking spray
1 pound large shrimp (about 24), shelled and deveined
2 tablespoons fresh lime juice
1 teaspoon cumin
1 ½ teaspoons chili powder
½ cup ketchup
2 tablespoons chopped cilantro
1 teaspoon ground coriander

In a small bowl, combine 1 tablespoon of the lime juice, ½ teaspoon of the cumin, the chili powder, ketchup, and cilantro. Stir to blend and refrigerate. Spray a broiler pan with vegetable cooking spray and preheat the broiler. In a large bowl, combine the remaining lime juice, cumin, and the ground coriander. Add the shrimp, tossing to coat. Broil the shrimp 4-6 inches form the heat for 3 minutes, turning them over midway. Let cool and transfer the shrimp to a medium bowl, cover and refrigerate until well chilled, about 30 minutes. Serve with the sauce.

SPICY SAUTEED SHRIMP WITH GARLIC, 105 calories (4 servings)

1 tablespoon extra-virgin olive oil
2 teaspoons butter
1 pound large shrimp (about 24), shelled and deveined
2 large garlic cloves, finely slivered or chopped
1/4 teaspoon crushed red pepper flakes
2 tablespoon lemon juice
1/8 teaspoon salt
1/8 teaspoon freshly ground black pepper

Heat the olive oil and butter in a large skillet over medium-high heat until the butter is melted. Add the shrimp, salt, and black pepper. Cook, stirring frequently, for 2-3 minutes. Stir in the garlic and pepper flakes and cook, stirring frequently, for 2 minutes, lowering the heat if the garlic begins to color. Remove from the heat and stir in the lemon juice. If desired, serve with parsley or basil sprinkles.

SHRIMP CREOLE, 110 calories (4 servings)

1 tablespoon extra-virgin olive oil
½ pound raw shrimp, peeled and deveined
½ tablespoon reduced-fat margarine
½ cup chopped onion
½ cup chopped celery
1/4 cup chopped green pepper
½ teaspoon thyme
1 small minced garlic clove
1 ½ cup chopped tomatoes
1 tablespoon tomato paste
1/8 cup fresh parsley
1/4 teaspoon salt
1/8 teaspoon freshly ground black pepper
4 large lettuce leaves

In a large skillet, heat margarine and olive oil. Add onion, celery, green pepper, thyme and garlic. Saute until the vegetables are soft and then add tomatoes, tomato paste, salt, and pepper and bring to a boil. Add shrimp and reduce heat. Simmer, stirring occasionally, for 30 minutes. Add parsley and simmer for 2 minutes. Serve over a lettuce leaf.

SHRIMP AND VEGETABLE GARLIC KABOBS, 65 calories (4 servings)

½ pound uncooked, peeled, deveined medium shrimp, thawed if frozen
1/4 cup lemon juice
1 tablespoon balsamic or red wine vinegar
4 large cloves garlic, thinly sliced
1 medium zucchini, sliced (2 cups)
1 large red bell pepper, cut into eighths
2 teaspoons sesame oil

Mix shrimp, lemon juice and vinegar in shallow glass dish, cover, and refrigerate 30 minutes. Remove shrimp from marinade and thread shrimp, garlic, zucchini and bell pepper alternately on each of eight 10- or 12-inch metal skewers. Brush with sesame oil. Set oven to broil and place kabobs on rack in broiler pan, 4-6 inches from heat. Broil for 8 minutes, turning once. Heat remaining marinade to boil and stir for 1 minute. Serve marinade with kabobs.

COMPONENT CALORIE COUNTS

1 ounce cheese (1 slice) averages 100 calories. Fat-free cheese averages 40 calories.

1 medium apple 81 calories
1 medium banana 105 calories
½ cup blackberries 37 calories, blueberries 41 calories, cantaloupe 29 calories, cherries 49 calories, cranberries 23 calories, gooseberries 33 calories, grapes 29 calories, raspberries 30 calories, strawberries 23 calories
½ medium grapefruit 37 calories
1 medium navel orange 65 calories
1 medium nectarine 67 calories
1 medium peach 37 calories
1 medium pear 98 calories
1 cup pieced pineapple 77 calories
1 medium plum 36 calories
1 medium tangerine 37 calories
1 cup cut watermelon 50 calories

½ bagel which averages 80 calories
1 slice cracked wheat 66 calories
1 slice french bread 81 calories
1 slice Italian bread 78 calories
1slice oatmeal bread 71 calories
1 pita pocket 106 calories
1 slice pumpernickel 82 calories
1 slice rye bread 66 calories
1 slice white bread 64 calories
1 slice whole wheat bread 61 calories
2 Fat-Free Nabisco Saltine crackers 24 calories

Yogurt can be a low-calorie option which adds more protein than vegetable dishes. There are many options for this product, and it is best to check the label to find those which offer 8 fluid ounce portions below 100 calories.

SNACKS

For snacks which have few calories when your hunger reaches a point where you just have to eat something, try the following:

1 cucumber	14 calories
1 stalk celery	10 calories
1 cup endive or lettuce dipped in vinegar	8 calories
1 dill pickle	6 calories
1 raw medium tomato	26 calories
1 cup sugar-free fruit-flavored gelatin	20 calories
1 large bottle of water	0 calories
1 large bottle of water with 3 tablespoons lemon juice	9 calories
1 cup black coffee	6 calories
1 cup black tea	2 calories
1 can diet beverage	2 calories

For snacks that have 100 calories when you are raising your intake to above 600 calories per day, try the following:

10-ounce glass of vanilla soymilk or skim milk
6 ounces nonfat plain yogurt
1 large hard-boiled egg
2/3 cup fat-free cottage cheese
1 large apple
1 banana
1 ½ cups fresh blueberries
1 small cantaloupe
1 2/3 cups grapes
1 large grapefruit
1 large orange
2 medium peaches
1 medium pear
2 ½ cups fresh strawberries
2 medium tangerines
3 large carrots or 25 baby carrots
2 whole cucumbers
3 large tomatoes
1 slice whole wheat or white bread toast with 1 teaspoon fruit preserves
½ whole wheat bagel with 1 teaspoon fat-free cream cheese
3 ½ (2 ½-inch) graham crackers
3 cups air-popped popcorn. Spray lightly with butter-flavored cooking spray and salt, or toss with soy sauce.
12 almonds

ENDNOTES

1   Milton, John, <u>Paradise Lost</u> (London: Longman, 1968), 11:471-474, 588. It is likely that Milton got his inspiration from the writings of Dr. Thomas Cogan (1545-1607), who published *The Haven of Health* in 1596. In that book, he claimed that the saying "more die by surfeit than by the sword" was true, and that moderation of food intake was necessary for good health. Chittenden, Russell H, <u>The Nutrition of Man</u> (New York: Frederick A. Stokes Company, 1907), 166-167.

2   Ibid., 270.

3   MacCuish, AC & Ford, MJ, "Dietary Management of Obesity and Obesity-Related Diseases," <u>The Treatment of Obesity</u>, edit. JF Munro (Lancaster, England: MTP Press Limited, 1979), 21.

4   Sinclair, Upton, <u>The Fasting Cure</u> (Mokelumne Hill, CA: Health Research, 1955), 51.

5   Heron, Melonie, "Deaths: Leading Causes for 2004," <u>National Vital Statistics Reports</u> 56(2007):8.

6   For the sake of convenience, I will use the term "obesity" to refer to both the "overweight" patient, who is generally defined as weighing 20% more than the "desirable weight," based on actuarial data of height and body weight, and the "severely overweight" patient, who is 40% more than is desirable. Council on Scientific Affairs, "Treatment of Obesity in Adults," <u>JAMA</u> 260(1988):2547.

7   "Overweight and Obesity," http://www.cdc.gov/nccdphp/dnpa/obesity.

8   "U. S. Obesity Rates Continue to Rise," <u>HemOnc Today</u> September 10, 2009:34.

9   Atkinson, Richard L, "Viruses as an Etiology of Obesity," <u>Mayo Clin Proc</u> 82(2007):1192-1198.

10   "Economic Impact of Obesity," http://obesityinamerica.org/economicimpact.html.

11   Andrew Renehan, PhD, senior lecturer at the University of Manchester in the United Kingdom, estimated that 124,000 new cancers would develop in Europe in 2008 due to BMI levels greater than 25. <u>HemOnc Today</u> October 25, 2009:19. Much of this increased risk of cancer has been attributed to the ingestion of animal products, and has led many proponents to promote a vegetarian diet, which has been shown to lessen the risk of cancer in many epidemiologic studies across the globe. See, Fuhrman, Joel, <u>Eat to Live: The Revolutionary Formula for Fast and Sustained Weight Loss</u> (New York: Little, Brown and Company, 2003), 81.

12   McGinnis, JM & Foege, WH, "Actual Causes of Death in the United States," <u>JAMA</u> 270(1993):2207-2212.

13   Marks, John & Schrijver, Jaap, "Reports Submitted on Behalf of the VLCD European Industry Group to the SCOOP Working Group on Very-Low Calorie Diets Between 1998 and 2001, Consolidated 2001," http://www. geocities.com/jmarkscam/marksandschrivjer.html?200720, 19.

14   "Economic Impact of Obesity,"
http://obesityinamerica.org/economicimpact.html.
15   Powers, Kinga A, Rehrig, Scott T & Jones, Daniel B, "Financial Impact
of Obesity and Bariatric Surgery," Med Clin N A (91(2007):324.
16   Fisler, Janis S & Drenick, Ernst J, "Starvation and Semistarvation Diets in
the Management of Obesity," Ann Rev Nutr 7(1987):479.
17   Rosenbaum, M, Leibel, RL & Hirsch, J, "Obesity," New Eng J Med
337(1997):396.
18   Stunkard, Albert J, Harris, Jennifer R, Pedersen, Nancy L & McClearn,
Gerald E, "The Body-Mass Index of Twins Who Have Been Reared Apart,"
New Eng J Med 322(1990):1483.
19   Farooqui, IS, Jebb, SA, Langmack G, Lawrence, E, Cheetham, CH,
Prentice, AM, Hughes, IA, McCamish, MA & O'Rahilly, S, "Effects of
Recombinant Leptin Therapy in a Child With Congenital Leptin Deficiency,"
New Eng J Med 341(1999):879-884.
20   Farooqui, I Sadaf, Wangensteen, Teresia, Collins, Stephan, Kimber,
Wendy, Matarese, Giuseppe, Keogh, Julia M, Lank, Emma, Bottomley, Bill,
Lopez-Fernandez, Judith, Ferraz-Amaro, Ivan, Dattani, Mehul T, Ercan, Oya,
Myhre, Anne Grethe, Retterstol, Lars, Stanhope, Richard, Edge, Julie A,
McKenzie, Sheila, Lessan, Nader, Ghodsi, Maryam, De Rosa, Veronica, Perna,
Francesco, Fontana, Silvia, Barroso, Ines, Undlien, Dag E & O'Rahilly,
Stephen, "Clinical and Molecular Genetic Spectrum of Congenital Deficiency
of the Leptin Receptor," New Eng J Med, 356(2007):237-247.
21   Licinio, J, Caglayan, S, Ozata, M, Yildiz, BO, de Miranda, PB, O'Kirwan,
F, Whitby, R, Liang, L, Cohen, P, Bhasin, S, "Phenotypic Effects of Leptin
Replacement on Morbid Obesity, Diabetes Mellitus, Hypogonadism, and
Behavior in Leptin-deficient Adults," Proc Natl Acad Sci 101(2002):4531-
4536.
22   Wren, AM, Seal, LJ, Cohen, MA, Brynes, AE, Frost, GS, Murphy, KG,
Dhillo, WS, Ghatei, MA, & Bloom, SR, "Ghrelin Enhances Appetite and
Increases Food Intake in Humans," J Clin Endocrinol Metab 86(2001):5992.
23   Cummings, DE, Weigle, DS, Frayo, RS, Breen, PA, Ma, MK, Dellinger,
EP, Purnell, JQ, "Plasma Gherlin Levels After Diet-Induced Weight Loss or
Gastric Bypass Surgery," New Eng J Med 346(2002):1623-1630.
24   Galland, Leo, The Fat Resistance Diet (New York: Broadway Books,
2005), 29.
25   Folin, Otto & Denis, W., "On Starvation and Obesity, With Special
Reference to Acidosis," J Biol Chem 21(1915):183.
26   Exod 34:28; Deut 9:9; 1 Kgs 19:8.
27   Matt 4:2.
28   The other 4 pillars include faith, prayer, charitable giving, and a
pilgrimage to Mecca. Fasting was used by Sufis who wished to hear the word
of God in their hearts, and "for some, two days and nights are enough; for still
others, a week; and some may need a full forty days." Sharafuddin Maneri,
"Letter 33," The Hundred Letters, transl. by Paul Jackson (New York: Paulist
Press, 1980), 129.

29   Benjamin D. Horne, PhD, director of cardiovascular and genetic epidemiology, Intermountain Medical Center, Salt Lake City, presented this data at the American Heart Association's Scientific Session 2007, Orlando, Fla., Nov 4-7, 2007. Http://www.webmd.com/heart-disease/news/20071106/fasting-may-cut-heart-risks?src=RSS_PUBLIC.

30   Folin & Denis, "On Starvation and Obesity, With Special Reference to Acidosis," 192. They also described a second patient with the same delay that was admitted for an infection of her leg. Ibid., 187.

31   Williams, Nutrition and Diet Therapy, 15.

32   Protein, on the average, is composed of 52% carbon, 23% oxygen, 16% nitrogen, 7% hydrogen, and 1% sulfur. It is our only source of nitrogen, and is therefore an essential component of our food supply. Lean meats and egg whites are composed primarily of protein, with other cuts of meat having variable amounts of fat. Carbohydrates consist of 44.4% carbon, 49.4% oxygen, and 6.2% hydrogen, while fats are 76.5% carbon, 11.5% oxygen, and 11.9% hydrogen. Although fats and carbohydrates undergo complete combustion to simple gaseous products when they are catabolized, proteins leave a nitrogen residue that must be excreted by the liver and kidneys.

33   Williams, Nutrition and Diet Therapy, 669.

34   Apfelbaum, Marian, Fricker, Jacques, & Igoin-Apfelbaum, Laurence, "Low- and Very-Low-Calorie Diets," Am J Clin Nutr 45(1987):1127.

35   Bray, George A, "Nutrient Balance and Obesity: An Approach to Control of Food Intake in Humans," Med Clin N A 73 (1989):31-33.

36   The increased health risk of the android pattern of fat distribution was first noted by Dr. Jean Vague, a French clinician from the University of Marseilles with a large obesity practice. Vague, J, "The Degree of Masculine Differentiation of Obesities: A Factor Determining Predisposition to Diabetes, Atherosclerosis, Gout, and Uric Calculous Disease," Am J Clin Nutr 4(1956):20-34.

37   Stefan, Norbert, Kantarzis, Konstantinos, Machann, Jurgen, Schick, Fritz, Thamer, Claus, Rittig, Kilian, Balletshofer, Bernd, Machicao, Fausto, Fritsche, Andreas, & Haring, Hans-Ulrich, "Identification and Characterization of Metabolically Benign Obesity in Humans," Arch Intern Med 168(2008):1615.

38   The problem affects 1 of every 20,000 births in the United States. Roe, Charles R., "MCAD: Medium Chain acyl CoA Dehydrogenase - Information for Clinicians," http://www. fodsupport.org/mcad.htm, 1-3.

39   The gene for MCAD is located on chromosome 1p31, and over 25 variants have already been described. "Definition of MCAD Deficiency," http://www.medterms.com/script/main/art.asp?articlekey=25325 1.

40   Thuillier, L, Rostane, H, Droin, V, Demaugre, F, Brivet, M, Kadhom, N, Prip-Buus, C, Gobin, S, Saudubray, JM, & Bonnefont, JP, "Correlation Between Genotype, Metabolic Data, and Clinical Presentation in Carnitine Palmitoyltransferase 2 (CPT2) Deficiency, Hum Mutat 21(2003): 493-501.

41   Dunne, Lavon J, Nutrition Almanac (New York: McGraw-Hill, Fifth Edition, 2002), 150.

42   Booyens, J, Louwrens, CC & Katzeff, IE, "The Role of Unnatural Dietary

Trans and Cis Unsaturated Fatty Acids in the Epidemiology of Coronary Artery Disease," Med Hypoth 25(1988):175-182.

43   Willett, WC & Ascherio, A, "Trans Fatty Acids: Are the Effects Only Marginal?" Am J Publ Hlth 85(1995):411-412.

44   "Trans Fat," http://en.widipedia.org/wiki/Trans_fat, 2.

45   Atkins, Robert C, Dr. Atkins' New Diet Revolution (New York: M. Evans & Company, Inc., 1992), 18.

46   Gardner, Christopher D, Kiazand, Alexandre, Alhassan, Sifiya, Kim, Soowon, Stafford, Randall S, Balise, Raymond R, Kraemer, Helena C & King, Abby C, "Comparison of the Atkins, Zone, Ornish, and LEARN Diets for Change in Weight and Related Risk Factors Among Overweight Premenopausal Women," JAMA 297(2007): 974

47   Fisler & Drenick, "Starvation and Semistarvation Diets in the Management of Obesity," 470.

48   Vasey, Christopher, The Detox Mono Diet: The Miracle Grape Cure and Other Cleansing Diets (Rochester, VT: Healing Arts Press, 2006), 34-35.

49   Sinclair, The Fasting Cure, 23-24. He referred to the fasting method as "Nature's safety-valve." Ibid., 25.

50   Shelton, Herbert M., Fasting Can Save Your Life, 36.

51   Cott, Allan, Fasting: The Ultimate Diet (New York: Bantam Books, Inc., 1975), 53.

52   Carrington, Hereward, Vitality, Fasting & Nutrition: A Physiological Study of the Curative Power of Fasting, Together With a New Theory of the Relation of Food to Human Vitality (Pomeroy, WA: Health Research, 1908), 94.

53   Dr. Tanner fell ill and fasted for 42 days in 1877, regaining so much of his health that he became an ardent proponent of the technique, undergoing another 40 day fast in 1880. "The Pioneers of Therapeutic Fasting in America," http://www.soilandhealth.org/02/0201hyglibcat/02197/hazzard/02017/hazzardc h1.html, 1-3. When he undertook his fast in 1880 in New York City, "no one could be found willing to believe that he could accomplish it." Gunn, Robert A., Forty Days Without Food!: A biopgraphy of Henry S. Tanner, M.D. (New York: Albert Metz & Co., 1880), 8.

54   Ehret, Arnold, Professor Arnold Ehret's Mucusless Diet Healing System (Cody, WY: Ehret Literature Publishing Co., 1953), 18, 24, 90.

55   Ehret, Arnold, Rational Fasting For Physical, Mental & Spiritual Rejuvenation (Dobbs Ferry, NY: Ehret Literature Publishing Co., Inc., 1926), 11.

56   Benedict, Francis Gano, A Study of Prolonged Fasting (Washington, DC: Carnegie Institute of Washington Publication No. 203, 1915).

57   Scientific papers studying the effects of starvation on metabolism began to appear in European and American journals in the 1890s. See Cathcart, EP, "On Metabolism during Starvation: I. Nitrogenous," J Physiol 35(1907):500-510.

58   Benedict, Francis. G, Miles, Walter R, Roth, Paul & Smith, H Monmouth, Human Vitality and Efficiency Under Prolonged Restricted Diet (Washington,

DC: Carnegie Institute of Washington No. 280, 1919).
59   Shelton, HM, Superior Nutrition (San Antonio: Willow Publishing, Inc., 1940), 134-137.
60   "Herbert M. Shelton," http.//en.wikepedia.org/wiki/Herbert_Shelton, 1.
61   Ibid.
62   Bloom, Walter Lyon, "Fasting as an Introduction to the Treatment of Obesity," Metab 8(1959):215.
63   Apfelbaum, Fricker, & Igoin-Apfelbaum, "Low- and Very-Low-Calorie Diets," Am J Clin Nutr 45(1987):1128.
64   "LeDiet," http://www.lediet.com/partners.html.
65   Shelton, Fasting Can Save Your Life, 24.
66   Stewart, WK & Fleming, Laura W, "Features of a Successful Therapeutic Fast of 382 Days' Duration," Postgrad Med J 49(1973):204, 206; Thomson, TJ, Runcie, J & Miller, V, "Treatment of Obesity by Total Fasting for up to 249 Days," Lancet 2(1966):992.
67   Stewart & Fleming, "Features of a Successful Therapeutic Fast of 382 Days' Duration," 207.
68   Strang, JM, McClugage, HB & Evans, FA, "Further Studies in the Dietary Correction of Obesity," Am J Med Sci 179(1930):693.
69   Howard, AN, "The Historical Development of Very Low Calorie Diets," Int J Obes 13(suppl.2, 1989):1-9.
70   Evans, Frank A & Strang, James M, "A Departure from the Usual Methods in Treating Obesity," Am J Med Sci 177(1929):342.
71   Simeons' concept was resurrected by Kevin Trudeau in his book Natural Cures "They" Don't Want You to Know About in 2005, eventually leading to action by the Federal Trade Commission (FTC) to restrict his promoting the book, and a conviction by a U. S. District Court in 2007 that Trudeau had misled thousands of consumers. "Trudeau," http://en.wikipedia.org/wiki/Kevin_Trudeau.
72   Bolinger, Robert E, Lukert, Barbara P, Brown, Robert W, Guevara, Lilia, & Steinberg, Ruth, "Metabolic Balance of Obese Subjects During Fasting," Arch Intern Med 118(1966):3-8.
73   Apfelbaum, M, Bostsarron, J, Brigant, L & Dupin, H, "Body Weight Loss Composition During Total Fast: Effects of a Protein Supplement," Gastroenterologia 108(1967):121-134.
74   Fisler & Drenick, "Starvation and Semistarvation Diets in the Management of Obesity," 467.
75   There are 9 amino acids which are considered essential because they must be provided by the food we eat: isoleucine, leucine, lysine, threonine, tryptophan, methionine, histidine, valine, and phenylalanine. Collagen protein is especially deficient in isoleucine and tryptophan, and contains only 36% of the essential amino acids present in soy-based protein. Fisler, Janis S, & Drenick, Ernst J, "Nitrogen Economy During Very Low Calorie Reducing Diets: A Comparison of Soy and Collagen Protein Supplements," Management of Obesity by Severe Caloric Restriction, edited by GL Blackburn & GA Bray (Littleton, MA: PSG Publishing Company, Inc., 1985), 93. The non-essential

amino acids, including alanine, arginine, asparagine, aspartic acid, cysteine, glutamic acid, glutamine, glycine, proline, serine, and tryosine, can all be created out of other chemicals in your body.

76   Amatruda, John M, Biddle, Theodore L, Patton, Mary L & Lockwood, Dean H, "Vigorous supplementation of a Hypocaloric Diet Prevents Cardiac Arrhythmias and Mineral Depletion," Am J Med 74(1983):1020. Linn prescribed a 600 calorie/day regimen based on his Prolinn drink which was a beef hide extract that did not meet the requirements of a high-quality protein as defined by the Food and Nutrition Board of the National Research Council. Newmark, Stephen R & Williamson, Beverly, "Survey of Very-Low-Calorie Weight Reduction Diets. II. Total Fasting, Protein-Sparing Modified Fasts, Chemically Defined Diets," Arch Intern Med 43(1983):1425.

77   They were first reported by the Center for Disease Control in 1977. "Deaths Associated with Liquid Protein Diets," Morbidity Mortality Weekly Reports 26(1977):383, 443.

78   There were 58 reports of deaths, but it was eventually determined that 17 of these were of sudden onset from a cardiac cause, possibly due to the diet itself. de Silva, Regis A., "Ionic, Catecholamine, and Dietary Effects on Cardiac Rhythm," Management of Obesity by Severe Caloric Restriction (Littleton, Mass: PSG Publishing Company, Inc., 1985), 195-196. It is believed that the reason for the deaths was cardiac arrest from ventricular fibrillation. Ibid., 198. The occurrence of ventricular fibrillation in patients undergoing liquid protein diets was initially reported in 1978. Singh, Bramah N, Gaarder, Thomas D, Kanegae, Thomas, Goldstein, Mark, Mongomerie, John Z & Mills, Harold, "Liquid Protein Diets and Torsade de Pointes," JAMA 240(1978):115-119; Brown, Jerry M, Yetter, Joseph F, Spicer, Melvin J & Jones, Jack D, "Cardiac Complications of Protein-Sparing Modified Fasting," JAMA 240(1978):120-122.

79   The Cambridge diet was devised by Alan Howard, PhD. Howard, AN, Grant, A, Edwards, O, Littlewood, ER, McLean, Baird, "The Treatment of Obesity by a Very-Low-Calorie Liquid-Formula Diet: An Inpatient/Outpatient Comparison Using Skimmed Milk as the Chief Protein Source," Int J Obes 2(1978):321-332.

80   New York Times November 24, 1988:B17.

81   Howard, Alan N, Letters, "The Cambridge Diet," JAMA 252(1984):897.

82   Hoffer, L John, Bistrian, Bruce R, & Blackburn, George L, "Composition of Weight Loss Resulting from Very Low Calorie Protein Only and Mixed Diets," Management of Obesity by Severe Caloric Restriction (Littleton, MA: PSG Publishing Company, Inc., 1985), 64.

83   Howard, AN, "The Development of a Very Low Calorie Diet: An Historical Perspective," Management of Obesity by Severe Caloric Restriction (Littleton, MA: PSG Publishing Company, Inc., 1985), 7-9.

84   Marks, & Schrijver "Reports Submitted on Behalf of the VLCD European Industry Group to the SCOOP Working Group on Very-Low Calorie Diets Between 1998 and 2001, Consolidated 2001," 10. The deaths that occurred with liquid protein diets were felt to "have no relevance to current VLCD."

Ibid.

85   Wadden, Thomas A, Van Itallie, Theodore B & Blackburn, George L, "Responsible and Irresponsible Use of Very-Low-Calorie Diets in the Treatment of Obesity," JAMA 263(1990):83

86   Carrington, Vitality, Fasting & Nutrition: A Physiological Study of the Curative Power of Fasting, Together With a New Theory of the Relation of Food to Human Vitality, 137.

87   Chittenden, The Nutrition of Man, 94-95.

88   "Louis Cornaro's Discourse on the Sober Life," http://www.wrf.org/men-women-medicine/louis-cornaro-discourse-sober-life.php.

89   McDougall, John, "A Brief History of Protein: Passion, Social Bigotry, Rats, and Enlightenment," http:// www.all-creatures.org/health/abrief-hi.html. Manual laborers in Europe and America during that era consumed, on average, 3400-5500 calories per day, with protein consumption of 115-189 gms. Chittenden, The Nutrition of Man, 155.

90   Ibid., 272. This could be provided by ½ pound of fresh lean beef for 308 calories, 9 eggs for 720 calories, 3/4 pound halibut steak for 423 calories, 2 quarts whole milk for 1300 calories, 5/6 pound uncooked oatmeal for 1550 calories, 1 pound uncooked macaroni for 1665 calories, 3/5 pound dried beans for 1125 calories, ½ pound dried peas for 827 calories, 2/3 pound almonds for 2020 calories, 10 pounds grapes or bananas for 4500 calories, 11 pounds lettuce for 990 calories, or 33 pounds apples for 9570 calories. Ibid., 274-275. Today, the recommended dietary allowance (RDA) for protein is 0.8 gm/kg/day for typical individuals, and 1.2-1.8 gm/kg/day for those performing regular, moderate- to high-intensity aerobic exercise. Rankin, Janet Walberg, "Role of Protein in Exercise," Clin Sprt Med 18(1999):500, 509.

91   The typical army ration consisted of beefsteak, potatoes and bread for breakfast, lunch and dinner, while the modified diet utilized fried hominy for breakfast, spaghetti, potatoes and bread for lunch, and fried bacon, sweet potatoes, bread and pudding for dinner. Brown, Goodwin, Scientific Nutrition Simplified: A Condensed Statement and Explanation for Everybody of the Discoveries of Chittenden, Fletcher, and Others (New York: Frederick A. Stokes Company, 1908), 32, 35-38.

92   Chittenden, The Nutrition of Man, 269.

93   Brown, Scientific Nutrition Simplified: A Condensed Statement and Explanation for Everybody of the Discoveries of Chittenden, Fletcher, and Others, 157-158.

94   Hazzard, Linda Burfield, Fasting For the Cure of Disease (New York: The Physical Culture Publishing Co., 4th ed., 1908), 18.

95   Brown, Scientific Nutrition Simplified: A Condensed Statement and Explanation for Everybody of the Discoveries of Chittenden, Fletcher, and Others, 3.

96   Ibid., 86.

97   "Roy Walford," http://en.wikipedia.org/wiki_Roy_Walford.

98   Delaney, Brian M & Walford, Lisa, The Longevity Diet: Discover Calorie Restriction - The Only Proven Way to Slow the Aging Process and Maintain Peak Vitality (New York: Marlowe & Company, 2005), xii.

99   Walford, Roy Y, The 120-Year Diet: How to Double Your Vital Years (New York: Four Walls Eight Windows, 2000); Walford, Roy L & Walford, Lisa, The Anti-Aging Plan: Strategies and Recipes For Extending Your Healthy Years (New York: Four Walls Eight Windows, 1994).

100   Meyerowitz, Steve, Juice Fasting & Detoxification (Summertown, TN: Book Publishing Company, 2002), 23. The theory for these complaints is that eliminating the intake of solid foods reduces the energy expended during the digestive process, allowing the body to focus on toxin excretion. In addition, juices contain many antioxidants and enzymes which are claimed to increase the excretion of toxins that lead to a variety of disease processes through a process known as "toxicosis," or toxemia. Advocates claim that "cancer cells, toxins, built-up chemicals, excess body fat, transformed fatty acids, impacted mucus in the bowel, sickness and disease are all dramatically impacted" by a juice-fast, including cancer, leukemia, arthritis, high blood pressure, kidney disorders, skin infections, liver disorders, alcoholism, and smoking. http://www.freedomyou.com/fasting_book/juice%20fasting.htm(2007), 2.

101   Ehret, Professor Arnold Ehret's Mucusless Diet Healing System, 43.

102   Gerson, Max, A Cancer Therapy: Results of Fifty Cases & the Cure of Advanced Cancer by Diet Therapy (New York: Whittier Books, 1958), 7.

103   Colborn, Theo, Dumanoski, Dianne & Myers, John Peterson, Our Stolen Future (New York: Plume Penguin Books, 1997), 139.

104   National Research Council, Environmental Epidemiology, Volume 1: Public Health and Hazardous Wastes (Washington, D.C.: National Academy Press, 1991), 26.

105   "Soaring Cancer Rates Blamed on Chemicals," http://mapcruzin.com/news/rtk031204a.htm.

106   Colborn, Dumanoski & Myers, Our Stolen Future, 106

107   Colbert, Don, Get Healthy Through Detox and Fasting (Lake Mary, FL: Siloam, 2006), 8-9.

108   "Get the Guide," http://www.foodnews.org/walletguide.php.

109   National Research Council, Environmental Epidemiology, Volume 1: Public Health and Hazardous Wastes, 173.

110   These patients were treated by a fast for 7-10 days approximately 26-35 months after being poisoned and many had a dramatic relief of their sufferings. Imamura, M & Tung, TC, "A Trial of Fasting Cure for PCB-poisoned patients in Taiwan," Am J Indus Med 5(1984):147-153.

111   Hubbard, L Ron, Clear Body, Clear Mind: The Effective Purification Program (Los Angeles: Bridge Publications, Inc., 1990), 13.

112   Ibid., 17, 19, 31, 44.

113   A special "Cal-Mag Formula" was taken 1-3 times daily by mixing 1 tablespoon of calcium gluconate in a normal-sized drinking glass, and adding ½ level teaspoon of magnesium carbonate and 1 tablespoon of cider vinegar. The mixture was stirred and ½ glass of boiling water was added to make the liquid

clear. The remainder of the glass was then filled with lukewarm or cold water. Ibid., 64. Patients also took multiple vitamin supplements, including niacin which was started at 100 mg per day and raised to as high as 5,000 mg per day. Ibid., 84, 88.

114 Ibid., 52-53.

115 Kirschner, HE, Live Food Juices (Monrovia, CA: H. E. Kirschner, 1957), 32-33, 37.

116 Ibid., 60-62.

117 Vasey, Christopher, The Acid-Alkaline Diet For Optimum Health (Rochester, VT: Healing Arts Press, 2003).

118 Vasey, The Detox Mono Diet: The Miracle Grape Cure and Other Cleansing Diets, 48.

119 Ibid., 120, 131.

120 Ibid., 52.

121 Burroughs, Stanley, The Master Cleanser (revised edition, 1993), 17.

122 "Stanley Burroughs," http://en.wikipedia.org/wiki/Stanley_Burroughs. See People v. Burroughs, 35 Cal.3d 824, (1984).

123 Buhner, Stephen Harrod, The Fasting Path: The Way to Spiritual, Physical, and Emotional Enlightenment (New York: Penguin Group (USA) Inc., 2003), 178-179.

124 Safron, Jeremy, The Fasting Handbook: Dining From an Empty Bowl (Berkeley: Celestial Arts, 2005), 14.

125 Campbell, T Colin & Campbell, Thomas M II, The China Study: The Most Comprehensive Study of Nutrition Ever Conducted and the Startling Implications for Diet, Weight Loss, and Long-term Health (Dallas: BenBella Books, Inc., 2006).

126 Ibid., 174.

127 Ibid., 83.

128 "Protein in Nutrition," http://en.wikipedia.org/wiki/Protein_in_nutrition, 2.

129 According to the USDA, the highest content of protein per measure of food is found in duck, chicken, halibut, salmon and turkey, with amounts averaging 41-51. On this same scale, soybeans contain 28.62, couscous 22.07, barley 19.82, lentils 17.86, bulgur 17.21, wheat flour 16.44, oat bran 16.24, and pinto beans 15.41, all greater than dark meat of a chicken 13.49, fish fillets 13.34, and ham 10.69. "USDA National Nutrient Database for Standard Reference, Release 20, http:///www.ars.usda.gov/Services/docs.htm?docid=8964, 3-5

130 Landsberg, Lewis & Young, James B, "Changes in Metabolic Rate: Role of Catecholamines and the Autonomic Nervous System," Management of Obesity by Severe Caloric Restriction (Littleton, Mass: PSG Publishing Company, Inc., 1985), 138.

131 Colbert, Get Healthy Through Detox and Fasting, 119.

132 Boschmann, Michael, Steiniger, Jochen, Hille, Uta, Tank, Jens, Adams, Frauke, Sharma, Arya M, Klaus, Susanne, Luft, Friedrich C. & Jordan, Jens, ""Water-Induced Thermogenesis," J Clin Endo Metab 88(2003):6015-6019.

133 This could be as high as 33-38 mm Hg systolic, beginning within 5 minutes after drinking started, and lasting for greater than 60 minutes. Jordan, Jens, Shannon, John R, Black, Bonnie K, Ali, Yasmine, Farley, Mary, Costa, Fernando, Diedrich, Andre, Robertson, Rose Marie, Biaggioni, Italo & Robertson, David, "The Pressor Response to Water Drinking in Humans," Circ 101(2000):504-509.

134 Dulloo, AG, Duret, C, Rohrer, D, Giradier, L, Mensi, N, Fathi, M, Chantre, P, Vandermander, J, "Efficacy of a Green Tea Extract Rich in Catechin Polyphenols and Caffeine in Increasing 24-h Energy Expenditure and Fat Oxidation in Humands," Am J Clin Nutr 70(1999):1040-5.

135 Fisler & Drenick, "Starvation and Semistarvation Diets in the Management of Obesity," 475.

136 "Omega-3 Fatty Acid," http://en.wikipedia.org/wiki/Omega-3_fatty_acid, 1-13.

137 The flaxseed oil diet originally proposed by Dr. Johanna Budwig (1908-2003) to treat cancer blends 2-5 tablespoons of flaxseed oil with 1 cup or low fat cottage cheese, a calorie intake of 400-760 calories.

138 Talbott, Shawn M, A Guide to Understanding Dietary Supplements (New York: The Haworth Press, 2003), 90.

139 Kalman, D, Colker, CM, Wilets, I, et.al., "The Effects of Pyruvate Supplementation on Body Composition in Overweight Individuals," Nutr 15(1999):337-340; Stank, RT, Tietze, D. & Arch, JE, "Body Composition, Energy Utilization, and Nitrogen Metabolism with a 4.25-MJ/d low-energy Diet Supplemented with Dihydroxyacetone and Pyruvate," Am J Clin Nutr 56(1992):630-635.

140 The ingestion of 6 grams of pyruvate daily for six weeks appeared to enhance weight loss and loss of body fat. Colker, CM, Antonio, & Kalman, DS, "Effects of Pyruvate on Body Composition and Lipid Levels of Overweight Individuals," J Am Diet Assoc 98(1998):s1, a50.

141 "Why You Should Consider Purifying Your Drinking Water," http://www.envirodoc.com/why-purify-drinking-water.htm.

142 Sodium nitroprusside reacts with acetoacetic acid to develop a color ranging from buff-pink to maroon. The strips do not react with acetone or beta-hydroxybutyric acid.

143 Apfelbaum, Fricker & Igoin-Apfelbaum, Laurence, "Low- and Very-Low-Calorie Diets," Am J Clin Nutr 45(1987):1128.

144 "Horace Fletcher," http://en.wikipedia.org/wiki/Horace_Fletcher, 1.

145 Burroughs, The Master Cleanser (revised edition, 1993), 21.

146 Airola, Paavo, How to Keep Slim, Healthy & Young With Juice Fasting (Phoenix: Health Plus, Publishers, 1971), 47. Glauber's salt has been used to treat acetaminophen overdose.

147 Walker, NW, Fresh Vegetable and Fruit Juices (Prescott, Arizona: Norwalk Press, 1970), 84.

148 "Detoxification," http://www.drlam.com/A3R_brief_in_doc_format/2002-No1-Detoxification.cfm, 7. Max Gerson (1881-1959), who developed the "Gerson

therapy" for the treatment of tuberculosis and cancer, popularized the use of coffee enemas in the treatment of cancer, in order to remove the pounds of feces which he believed was one of the causes of cancer. He gave enemas every four hours, along with 2 tablespoons of castor oil and a castor oil enema every other day. The coffee enema was prepared by boiling 3 tablespoons of ground coffee in one quart of water for 3 minutes. Gerson, A Cancer Therapy: Results of Fifty Cases & the Cure of Advanced Cancer by Diet Therapy, 190-191, 194.

149 Shelton, Fasting Can Save Your Life, 68.

150 Buchinger, Otto HF, About Fasting, transl. Geoffrey A Dudley (Wellingborough, Northamptonshire: Thosons Publishers Unlimited, 1961), 37, 45.

151 Bragg, Paul C & Bragg, Patricia, The Miracle of Fasting: Proven Throughout History for Physical, Mental & Spiritual Rejuvenation (Santa Barbara: Health Science).

152 Hendler, Rosa & Bonde, Alfons A III, "Very-Low-Calorie Diets with High and Low Protein Content: Impact on Triiodothyronine, Energy Expenditure, and Nitrogen Balance," Am J Clin Nutr 48(1988):1242.

153 It has been hypothesized that this may be due to nocturnal elevations of leptin hormone. Van Cauter, Eve, Polonsky, Kenneth S & Scheen, Andre J, "Roles of Circadian Rhythmicity and Sleep in Human Glucose Regulation," Endo Rev 18(1997):718.

154 Wing, RR, "Physical Activity in the Treatment of Adulthood Overweight and Obesity: Evidence and Research Issues," Med Sci Sports Exercise 31(Suppl 11, 1999): S547-S552.

155 Apfelbaum, Fricker, & Igoin-Apfelbaum, "Low- and Very-Low-Calorie Diets," Am J Clin Nutr 45(1987):1132.

156 Wadden, Van Itallie & Blackburn, "Responsible and Irresponsible Use of Very-Low-Calorie Diets in the Treatment of Obesity," JAMA 263(1990):83. In the 461 studies reviewed by the VLCD European Industry Group, representing the results in 52,783 subjects, 33% used the diet for under 4 weeks, and 67% for 4 weeks or more. Marks & Schrijver, "Reports Submitted on Behalf of the VLCD European Industry Group to the SCOOP Working Group on Very-Low Calorie Diets Between 1998 and 2001, Consolidated 2001," 24.

157 Genuth, Saul M, Castro, Jamie H, & Vertes, Victor, "Weight Reduction in Obesity by Outpatient Semistarvation," JAMA 230 (1974):987.

158 Ibid., 84.

159 Wadden, Thomas A, "Treatment of Obesity by Moderate and Severe Caloric Restriction. Results of Clinical Research Trials," Ann Intern Med 119(1993):689.

160 Davis, JM, et al., "Weight Control and Calorie Expenditure: Thermogenic Effects of Pre-Prandial and Post-Prandial Exercise," Addic Behav 14(1989):347-351.

161 "Fasting for Health," http://www.geocities.co.jp/Beautycare-Venus/2032/english/paper/.html, 1.

162 "Life Extension Vitamins,"

http://www.lifeextensionvitamins.com/faandcarewid.html, 3.

163   Foster-Powell, Kaye, Holt, Sussana HA, & Brand-Miller, Janette C, "International Table of Glycemic Index and Glycemic Load Values: 2002," Am J Clin Nutr 76(2002): 5-56.

164   Shelton, Herbert M, Willard, Jo & Oswald, Jean A, The Original Natural Hygiene Weight Loss Diet Book (New Canaan, CT: Keats Publishing, Inc., 1986), 100.

CPSIA information can be obtained at www.ICGtesting.com
Printed in the USA
LVOW030448160911

246546LV00012B/59/P